The Plant-Based Anti-Inflammatory Cookbook

Delicious Whole-Food Recipes to Reduce Inflammation and Promote Health

Linda Tyler, creator of
GraciousVegan.com

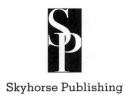

Skyhorse Publishing

Skyhorse Publishing books may be purchased in bulk at special discounts for sales promotion, corporate gifts, fund-raising, or educational purposes. Special editions can also be created to specifications. For details, contact the Special Sales Department, Skyhorse Publishing, 307 West 36th Street, 11th Floor, New York, NY 10018 or info@skyhorsepublishing.com.

Skyhorse® and Skyhorse Publishing® are registered trademarks of Skyhorse Publishing, Inc.®, a Delaware corporation.

Visit our website at www.skyhorsepublishing.com.

10 9 8 7 6 5 4 3

Library of Congress Cataloging-in-Publication Data is available on file.

Cover design by Kai Texel
Cover photo by Linda Tyler

Print ISBN: 978-1-5107-7735-4
Ebook ISBN: 978-1-5107-7736-1

Printed in China

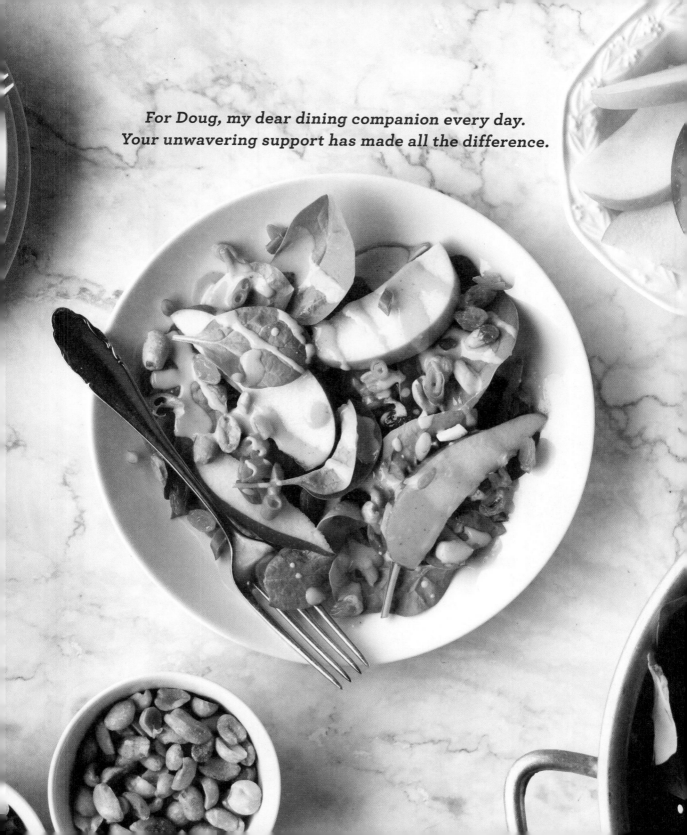

For Doug, my dear dining companion every day.
Your unwavering support has made all the difference.

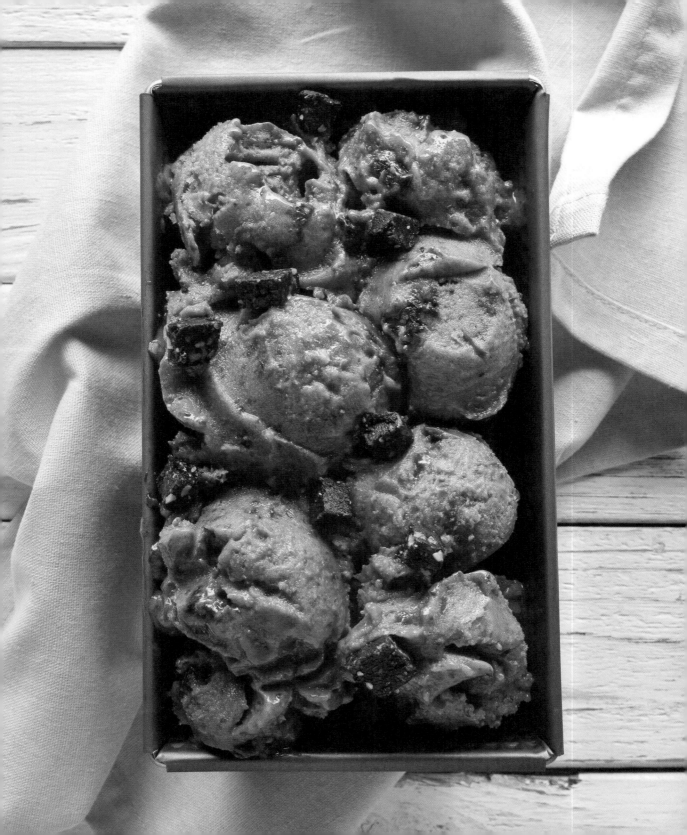

Contents

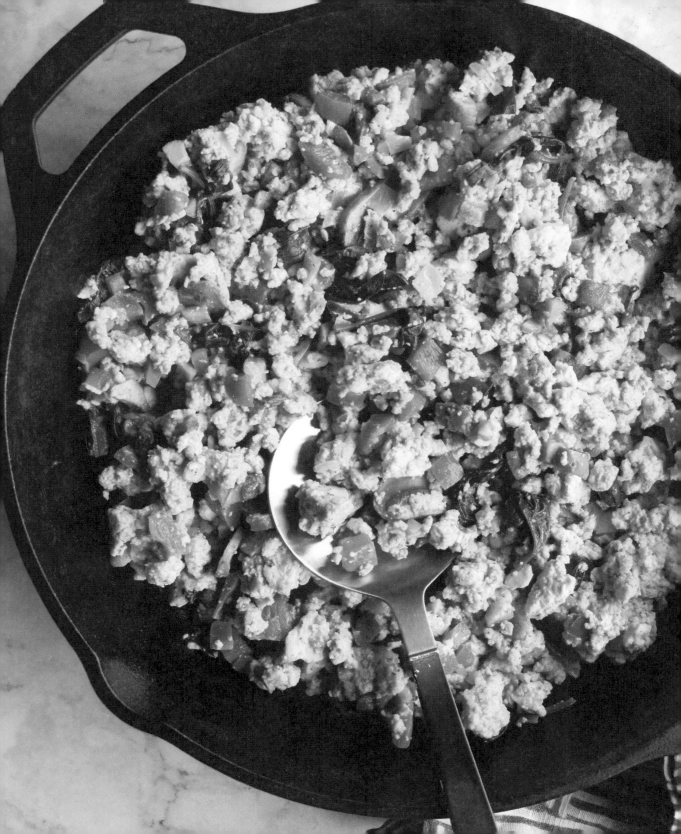

Introduction

Hippocrates said "let food be thy medicine." Sounds good, yes? Ask people if they agree, and many would say yes. But we know from grocery store sales, restaurant menus, and fast food choices that most people don't eat like they believe it. Some don't have the means to choose and buy only healthy foods. Some don't have the knowledge. And food's other roles as comfort, connection, tradition, reward, and recreation often triumph over food's medicinal potential.

My family tree includes a wide array of deadly diseases—cancer, heart attack, congestive heart disease, stroke, and Parkinson's. These are just the ones that killed my parents and grandparents. I want to use food as medicine to help me avoid an early death.

But mere survival or longevity isn't the goal. I want to thrive. I want to hike Yosemite Falls in my seventies. I'd love to run the Portland Half Marathon into my eighties (when showing up truly is 90 percent of success). I want to still be playing the piano in my nineties. I want to work in my garden, laugh with family and friends, write, take photos, and teach for many more years.

As it happens, the diseases in my family tree and the conditions that hold back an energetic life have one thing in common: inflammation. Chronic inflammation can create an environment that allows diseases and disorders to start, grow, and flourish. By focusing on a diet that science has shown to be most effective for lowering inflammation, I'm hoping to live my best life and hold off the diseases that brought down my parents and grandparents too early in their lives.

A plant-based diet is an excellent way to calm inflammation and lower our risk of chronic diseases. A systematic review and meta-analysis of forty research studies found that vegan- and vegetarian-based dietary patterns were associated with lower concentrations of inflammation markers in the blood compared with non-vegetarian diets.[1]

1 Joel C. Craddock, Elizabeth P. Neale, Gregory E. Peoples, Yasmine C. Probst, "Vegetarian-Based Dietary Patterns and their Relation with Inflammatory and Immune Biomarkers: A Systematic Review and Meta-Analysis," *Advances in Nutrition*, Volume 10, Issue 3, May 2019, Pages 433–451, https://doi.org/10.1093/advances/nmy103.

There's a lot to unpack and define about how a plant-based diet fights inflammation, and I'll do that in the following chapters.

This cookbook is for those who want to calm chronic inflammation with food, but not at the expense of enjoyment or satisfaction. I've developed the recipes in this cookbook to be tasty and filling in addition to being anti-inflammatory. As you'll see in the next chapter, a plant-based diet generally and certain plant foods specifically are linked to lower levels of chronic inflammation and can go a long way toward decreasing inflammation and lowering the risk of related diseases.

The next chapter offers recommendations on cooking techniques, equipment, and meal prep approaches to help make this kind of cooking feasible for those who are new to healthy plant-based cooking and especially those who have a busy life and need as many shortcuts and efficiencies as possible.

The eighty recipes that follow encompass my favorite cuisines and most beloved ingredients. The goal of each dish is to be delicious in its own right, not just "okay for a plant-based recipe." I believe we can have it all—pleasure, satisfaction, and lower inflammation—on a plant-based diet, and I hope that some of these recipes become lifelong favorites for you.

If you suffer from inflammation caused by allergies or an autoimmune disease, the plant-based approach described here and reflected in my recipes could go a long way toward helping calm the swelling and pain you experience. However, you may need to work with a dietician or doctor to uncover other food sensitivities or triggers that exacerbate your condition. In some cases, if diet alone does not relieve inflammation, medication may be needed as well. I've provided several resources that offer in-depth nutritional information for autoimmune conditions in the Resources and Deep Dives chapter (page 267).

My Journey to Healthy Plant-Based Cooking

When I was nineteen, I joined a big evangelical church in Southern California. One Sunday, I saw a flyer in the church's bulletin about their annual potluck picnic, including pie- and cake-baking contests. I definitely wanted to go to the picnic but didn't even consider entering a competition. Me? Against all those experienced church-lady bakers? The idea was so ludicrous it didn't even cross my mind.

Several weeks later I went to the picnic and took my favorite carrot cake, which I'd made many times before from a favorite family recipe. When I dropped the cake off at the dessert table, I told the person that the cake was a potluck dish, not an entry for the contest. A couple hours later, I was deep into conversation with friends when the head judge of the baking contest took to the microphone. After the preliminaries, which I barely paid attention to, I heard him announce that the blue ribbon for Best Cake went to Linda Tyler. Whaaaa? How could that be? I hadn't even entered my cake into the contest. My friends pushed me forward, and I stumbled through the crowd of smiling faces to pick up my ribbon. Me? My carrot cake? Wow, this required a rethink.

Maybe I should have applied for culinary school right then and there. But I'm not even sure I knew what culinary school was back then. I was majoring in music at the University of California, Riverside, near where I grew up, thinking I would become a college music professor if I couldn't make it as a concert pianist. Working as a culinary professional never occurred to me until much later in life.

But I kept cooking. I'd been cooking and baking since I was a little girl—in fact, I can't remember *not* cooking and *not* helping my mom in the kitchen. My little sister and I spent a lot of time there, the central gathering place in our small house. Sometimes we cooked with our mom by choice—we liked Saturdays, "baking day"—and sometimes we were there by fiat, our parents being big believers in chores.

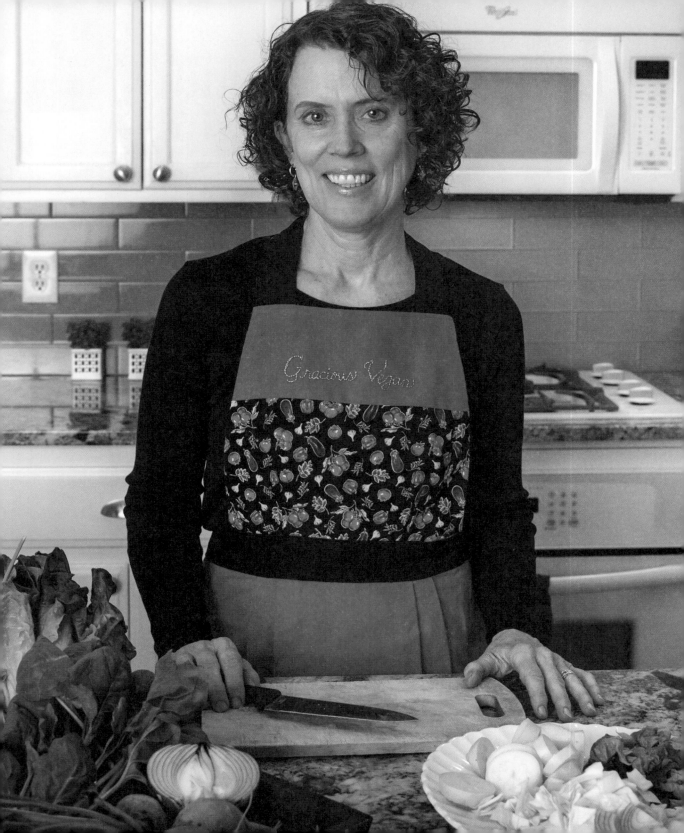

I decided to go vegetarian when I was twenty in an attempt to lose the weight I'd gained from dorm food. Within months I developed a strong distaste for meat. I never looked back after I learned about the cruel system of factory farming. When I got my own apartment and started cooking for myself, I latched onto the only vegetarian cookbook I could find at the time, *Diet for a Small Planet.* For a few years I relied on Frances Moore Lappé's protein-packed entrees along with nonmeat recipes from Betty Crocker.

Several years later, when I was in graduate school at Princeton studying music history, I fell in love with Mollie Katzen's *Moosewood Cookbook.* Mollie expanded my horizons more than any other cookbook writer before or since. I started cooking with ingredients my mother never used: real garlic, fresh ginger, mushrooms, feta cheese, bulgur, green onions, winter squash, eggplant, fresh basil, and so much more.

In 2010, several decades after I'd become a vegetarian, an issue of *VegNews* magazine arrived with articles on the dairy and egg industries. I'd been blind to the cruelties of milk and egg farms until then and quickly realized I had to go vegan. I gave myself a year to make the transition, but it only took a couple of months—the vision of miserable hens and dairy cows haunted me. I decided I could give up eggs, milk, half-and-half, and cheese for them.

That meant another reinvention of my cooking. Almost all of my go-to recipes for dinner with my husband contained cheese. And I'd always used eggs in baked goods. Back to the drawing board. I had to learn about flaxseed meal, chia seeds, and other new baking ingredients. I rebuilt my cake and pie repertory, but it took a while to re-earn the oohs and ahhs. (Yes, I finally tinkered my way to a perfect vegan carrot cake.)

My final eating and cooking transformation began in 2015 when I attended the Vegetarian Summerfest in Johnstown, Pennsylvania. There I discovered healthy plant-based eating, which was coming into its own at the time. I heard Dr. Michael Greger and Dr. T. Colin Campbell speak; I saw cooking demos by Chef AJ and ate meals prepared by Mark Reinfeld; I went to breakout sessions led by Julieanna Hever and other dieticians. I'd come to the conference for animal welfare discussions but left committed to unprocessed, oil-free, sugar-free cooking and eating. I realized I could be kind to animals and the environment while eating the healthiest diet on the planet.

In the kitchen, the transformation to a healthy plant-based diet led me to water sauté my onions and garlic, use tahini and roasted sesame paste instead of oil, drizzle balsamic vinegar on foods I'd never drizzled anything on before, blend salad dressings without oil, and rely on the sweetness of dates instead of sugar. I found great plant-based recipes on the internet, but I always adapted them. And I didn't want to give up on the dishes I'd come to love. I fiddled with and tweaked meat and dairy recipes from my formerly favorite cookbooks and websites—especially Ina Garten, Deborah Madison, and *NYT Cooking*. Gradually I had notebooks full of my own creations, and when I shared them, others loved them too.

All of the cooking in my thirties, forties, and fifties was done while I worked full-time for an education company. I taught myself a lot of meal prep tricks, like chopping vegetables in the morning before I left and making enough dinner for leftovers so I could get two dinners out of any dish I cooked. I often spent half a day each weekend in the kitchen. I can relate to having to squeeze cooking into a busy schedule, and this cookbook was written with that in mind.

Once I went to part-time work, I started my own website and volunteered to demonstrate plant-based recipes in the Portland area, my new home base. A few years after that, I began teaching plant-based cooking classes for Portland Community College and Mt. Hood Community College. I also started to coach people one-on-one who wanted to go plant-based or eat healthier. There's nothing like hearing from a student how much they and their family enjoyed a recipe. It's like winning a blue ribbon all over again.

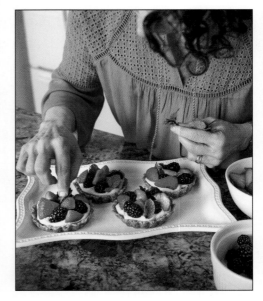

I've learned a lot about specific plant-based foods and how they can improve our health through my volunteer work over the last eight years with Dr. Michael Greger's Nutrition Facts organization. Through their work I came to understand how dangerous chronic inflammation can be to our health. Because of the information on their site and Dr. Greger's books *How Not to Die* and *How Not to Diet,* I came to understand the basics about chronic inflammation. I've done much more research since then and have gradually steered my own eating and recipes toward anti-inflammatory foods.

My love of cooking and commitment to health go hand in hand. None of us have to choose between what's good for us and what tastes good. The transition to a plant-based anti-inflammatory diet may take months or years, but the effort is worth it. Studies show over and over again that quality of life for most people is greater with a plant-based diet.

Whatever your family tree, wherever you are in your eating habits, however your body is afflicted or not, I hope your journey toward more plant-based eating—or, if you're already plant-based, your journey toward more focused anti-inflammatory eating—is a delicious, satisfying, and joyful one.

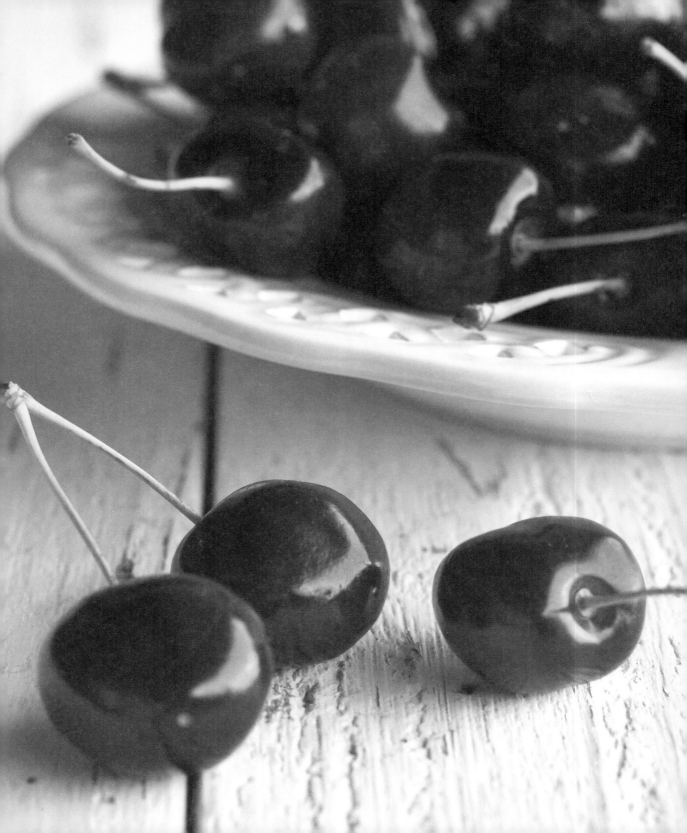

PART I
Cooking to Calm Inflammation

Lowering Chronic Inflammation through Diet

Over the many months while I was researching for this book, I was also raising a new rambunctious kitten, a Russian Blue named Serge. No matter how careful I was, Serge occasionally landed a scratch on my arm or a bite on my leg. I'd often have multiple scratches and bites in different stages of the healing process: bleeding, swollen redness, scabbing, and faint scarring.

I realized at some point during my research that my body's way of dealing with Serge's attacks had a direct connection to the type of chronic inflammation that's linked to serious disease and pain. I finally saw how it all fit together. That's why I think it's important to go back to the actual source of inflammation to better understand it.

Our Immune System—the Source of Inflammation

To understand what chronic inflammation is, I had to relearn the immune system, since it's the immune system that inflicts inflammatory damage.

While the purpose of our immune systems is to monitor what enters our bodies, deal with harmful invaders, and start the healing process, unfortunately, the immune system's reaction to certain substances or irregularities in the body can make things worse.

The major actors of the immune system are not organs, but billions of immune cells and trillions of proteins positioned all over our body, constantly on the alert and ready to be activated at a nanosecond's notice.

Immune cells—also called leukocytes or white blood cells—are the most critical players in the immune system. There are thousands of different types of immune cells, with different roles, triggers, and secretions. The other major players in the immune system are trillions of proteins, the most numerous of which are cytokines. Cytokines serve as messengers for the immune system. Immune cells secrete cytokines, which then signal other immune cells to come and help address a situation.

While immune cells and proteins can travel through the body via blood and lymph vessels, most of them are stationed in tissues or mucous layers, especially where germs and toxins are liable to enter the body. Researchers estimate that 70–80 percent of immune cells are positioned in or near the digestive system, and many others reside in the skin. The gut and skin are the locations where the outer world is most likely to get in.

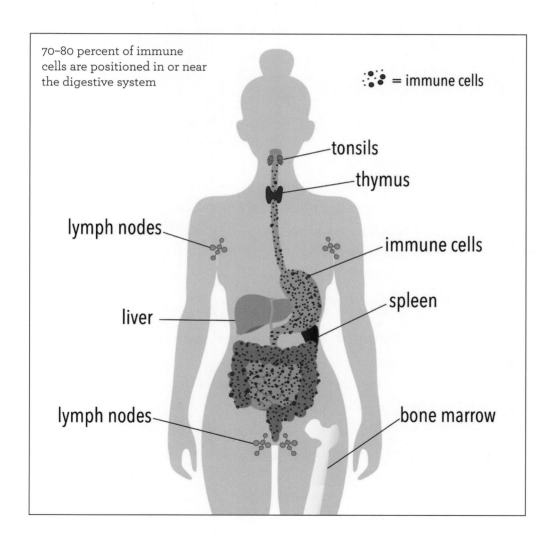

The organs and other parts of the immune system play mostly supporting roles to the trillions of immune cells and proteins. The liver, spleen, thymus, bone marrow, tonsils, and lymph system make possible the birth, development, storage, adaptation, and travel of the immune cells.

The Immune Response

Immune cells' reaction to a perceived enemy is called "the immune response." The immune response starts when local immune cells detect an irregularity and send out chemical signals. Blood flow to the area increases. Blood vessels swell and become more permeable, allowing immune and other cells, proteins, and fluids to cross more easily from the bloodstream into tissues. Immune cells begin to attack suspicious bodies, release chemicals to call for more immune cells, and clean up damaged tissue and waste. Many different types of immune cells and proteins work together in complex ways to carry out these tasks.

This immune response is much the same regardless of the trigger, location in the body, type of perceived threat, or scale of the threat; that is, blood flow and fluids rise, vessels swell and become more permeable, immune cells attack, proteins carry messages, and other immune cells dispose of dead tissues and debris. Whether the immune response lasts only a few days (called "acute inflammation") or for weeks, months, or years (called "chronic inflammation"), the immune response continues with virtually the same mechanisms.

Consequence of the Immune Response: Inflammation

The immune response has consequences for the body. Even though the response is usually beneficial, often lifesaving, in most cases it brings aftereffects. These consequences of the immune response are together called inflammation.

Since at least ancient Roman times, medical professionals have recognized the major signs of inflammation, even though the complexities of the immune process were not clear to them. The four cardinal signs of inflammation are:

- **Redness**—caused by swollen blood vessels
- **Heat**—caused by increased blood flow

- **Swelling**—caused by extra blood and fluid flowing into the affected area
- **Pain**—caused by swelling and certain chemicals released by immune cells during their response

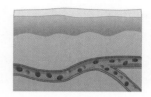

The Romans' description has stood the test of time, and most of us immediately recognize these sensations from times when we've been injured, fought off a virus, scratched an insect bite, or suffered from allergies. See the diagram here for a depiction of the immune response and the four signs of the inflammatory consequences.

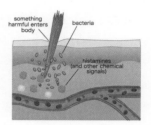

The Most Common Inflammation-Related Conditions

The immune response and consequent inflammation occur in many different circumstances. The following list includes the most common conditions that involve immune system activity:

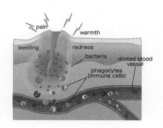

Injury

When we get a scratch, cut, fracture, broken bone, or other injury, immune cells work to catch and kill foreign invaders or toxins, dispose of dead tissue and debris, and start the healing process. This immune response usually

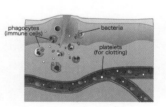

results in inflammation in and around the injured area: swelling, redness, heat, and pain.

Infection

After exposure to a virus or bacteria, immune cells mobilize and attack the invaders, with consequent inflammation in the form of a swollen sore throat, muscle aches, and congestion. Some infections can become chronic, and in the worst cases, the immune system is unable to contain the infection.

Allergies

In some people, the immune system mistakes otherwise harmless substances like pollen, peanuts, milk, or cat dander as dangerous invaders. The immune cells mount a response, and the sufferer feels the inflammation consequences—redness, swelling, pain—until the immune attack subsides or is countered by medication.

Autoimmune conditions

When the immune system attacks the body's own organs or tissues, mistaking them for dangerous substances, we call this an autoimmune condition. We still don't know enough about whether genetics, infections, toxins, an unhealthy gut, or something else causes or triggers most cases of autoimmune conditions, but the inflammation that comes from constant immune cell reactions can be very painful and destructive. Some of the most common autoimmune conditions are rheumatoid arthritis, Lupus, Crohn's disease, multiple sclerosis, type 1 diabetes, ulcerative colitis, Graves' disease, Hashimoto's thyroiditis, and celiac disease.

Other inflammatory-related conditions

When the immune system is having trouble clearing out invaders in a particular organ or body part, or is triggered in some other way, severe localized inflammation can come as a result of the immune cells and proteins attempting to gain the upper hand. Inflammatory conditions of this kind usually include the suffix "-itis," such as tonsillitis, laryngitis, bronchitis, and appendicitis. There are dozens of "-itis" conditions, too numerous to name here, that are all characterized by inflammatory consequences—swelling, redness, heat, and pain.

Low-grade internal inflammation (also known as "chronic inflammation")

Immune cells can wage fights on the cholesterol that lines coronary arteries, cells or molecules released from excess body fat, unstable or toxic substances in tissues, and compounds that enter the bloodstream from what we eat. These fights can result in a type of constant, internal, low-grade inflammation in our blood, tissues, and organs that we might not be able to feel, but can have harmful effects on our health, such as swelling, an excess of blood and fluids, and sometimes damage to healthy tissue.

Chronic Inflammation's Link to Deadly Diseases

Low-grade chronic inflammation appears to play a central role in some of the deadliest diseases on the planet. A constant state of inflammation makes us more vulnerable to serious diseases by creating the conditions in which diseases can emerge and grow. Often those diseases, in turn, can crank up the level of inflammation.

Chronic inflammation appears to be interconnected with the following major diseases:

Cardiovascular disease

Inflammation and cardiovascular disease are so often found together that doctors who suspect a patient might have early cardiovascular disease typically order a blood test that measures levels of inflammation markers in the blood, including C-reactive protein, interleukin-6, and/or fibrinogen. There's still a lot of research to be done to find the exact cause-and-effect links at play between heart disease and inflammation, but we do know that immune cells can react to plaque on artery walls once cholesterol begins to accumulate, swelling the artery walls and creating a constant state of inflammation. Sometimes the level of immune cell activity actually loosens a patch of built-up plaque, which can trigger blood clots with the potential to cause heart attacks or strokes.

Type 2 diabetes

Chronic inflammation can thwart cells' ability to absorb insulin, the hormone that helps cells use and store blood sugar. This "insulin resistance" is at the core of type 2 diabetes. Once cells slow down on sugar absorption, the sugar remains in the blood, which can lead to heart or kidney disease or problems with vision or sores. Unfortunately, insulin resistance can spawn more inflammation, creating a vicious cycle that often worsens diabetes and leads to ever-declining health.

Cancer

Cancer starts with a genetic mutation within a cell. Chronic inflammation can contribute to an environment of oxidative stress and DNA damage that can encourage genetic mutations and help new cancer cells grow. In addition, researchers have found that immune cells are often present within tumors and help the tumors grow. Although immune cells often fight cancer cells, they also appear in some cases to promote all phases of cancer, from early mutation through tumor growth and even late-stage metastasis.

Alzheimer's disease

Chronic inflammation can even take a toll on neurons in the brain. Studies have found that people with chronic inflammation during middle age have a greater risk of developing Alzheimer's disease and dementia later in life.

The last few decades of research have shown again and again that inflammation is a big risk factor for major diseases and premature death.

What Causes Low-Grade Chronic Inflammation?

Chronic inflammation can develop in our bodies for the following reasons, some of which we can control and some we can't:

Unhealthy environment

Chronic inflammation can grow when the immune system tries to fight off toxins (mold, heavy metals, pesticides, etc.) or pollutants (ozone, nitrogen dioxide, smoke, etc.) that get into the body. If exposure to noxious substances continues, the immune cells keep trying to fight them off, and healthy tissue becomes collateral damage in the battle.

Age

Chronic inflammation tends to rise as we get older. This increase may be due to aging cells, which secrete compounds that the immune system reacts to, or it could come from other age-related changes, like added body fat. As we age, we are more prone to unwanted inflammation.

Excess weight

Extra pounds are not—unfortunately—just dead weight. Fatty tissue actually secretes cytokines and other compounds into the body that trigger immune cells to mount their response, which generates inflammatory consequences. In another cruel twist, both weight gain and chronic inflammation can impair the brain's responsiveness to the hormone leptin, which tells the brain when we don't need to keep eating. Leptin resistance means we have more hunger pangs, making weight loss even harder.

Smoking
Certain chemicals in cigarette smoke generate unstable molecules called free radicals that can damage the lining of the lungs, which in turn trigger immune response and inflammation.

Stress
In people with high cortisol levels from stress, the immune system can become overactivated and out of balance. Our immune response can be triggered, with inflammatory results throughout the body. Stress also creates more free radicals in the blood that can damage cells and create a state of oxidative stress, setting off more immune responses.

Pro-inflammatory diet
We'll cover this topic in detail below.

We can't control our age or exposure to dangerous chemicals, but we can act on how we eat, exercise, sleep, deal with stress, and whether or not we smoke.

The rest of this chapter will focus on what we eat. It explains how diet can help calm inflammation and make us less vulnerable to its risks. We'll cover the foods to avoid because they increase inflammation and the foods to eat more of because they reduce it. Eating an inflammatory-calming diet can go a long way toward controlling the fire of inflammation, lowering our risk of deadly diseases, and helping us feel better.

The Role Diet Plays in Chronic Inflammation
A systematic review and meta-analysis of forty research studies found that diet can have a strong effect on our level of low-grade chronic inflammation and related disease.[2]

---

2   Joel C. Craddock, Elizabeth P. Neale, Gregory E. Peoples, Yasmine C. Probst, "Vegetarian-Based Dietary Patterns and their Relation with Inflammatory and Immune Biomarkers: A Systematic Review and Meta-Analysis," *Advances in Nutrition*, Volume 10, Issue 3, May 2019, Pages 433–451, https://doi.org/10.1093/advances/nmy103.

People who eat a vegan diet have lower levels of inflammatory markers in their blood on average than omnivores, pescatarians, and vegetarians. Vegans also have fewer cases of inflammation-related conditions like cardiovascular disease, type 2 diabetes, cancer, and Alzheimer's. Researchers have found that a high intake of fruit, vegetables, whole grains, and legumes is the key to lowering the body's inflammation. Some plant-based foods are especially good at lowering inflammation. We'll cover these at the end of this chapter.

A meat-based or "Western" diet brings greater risk of chronic inflammation. Most processed food, prepackaged foods, fast foods, meats, dairy, and restaurant meals contain nutrients that induce excess immune response with a consequence of ongoing inflammation. The good news, though, is that inflammation can be lowered when these foods are replaced with whole plant-based foods.

Foods That Increase Inflammation

The primary nutritional culprits in typical Western diets are saturated fats, endotoxins, and rapidly digested carbohydrates (e.g., white sugar and white flour). We need to minimize our intake of these compounds to lower chronic inflammation.

Saturated fat

Saturated fats appear to increase immune cell response and inflammation in several ways, including by increasing permeability of the gut wall, which allows toxins into the blood that immune cells react to; by increasing oxidative stress, which activates the immune system; and by degrading the balance of healthy and unhealthy bacteria in the gut microbiome, which also activates the immune response.

Endotoxins

Endotoxins contain lipopolysaccharides, which are powerful activators of the immune system. Endotoxins are released when certain kinds of bacteria (called gram-negative bacteria) die. These bacteria are most numerous in animal-based foods.

Refined sugar and grains

Elevated blood sugar levels, which can come from meals high in refined sugars and grains, lead to an increase in free radicals, causing oxidative stress and increased immune response.

Unfortunately, a large portion of the typical Western diet contains these pro-inflammatory culprits. Replacing familiar foods in the standard American diet with healthy plant-based alternatives can take time, effort, and perseverance. Even vegans who eat a lot of processed vegan foods with high levels of saturated fat and refined sugars and grains are risking an increase in their inflammation levels. The effort to make a transition to anti-inflammatory foods, though, can lead to a big payoff in longevity and vitality.

Foods to Minimize
Restaurant, takeout, and fast food

Who doesn't love the convenience of having someone else cook and clean up? Unfortunately, restaurant foods tend to be high in pro-inflammatory saturated fat, endotoxins, and refined sugars and grains.

- Breakfasts with eggs and side dishes
- Cheesy-buttery entrees
- Coffee beverages with whole milk, cream, or whipped cream
- Fried foods
- Hamburgers, including fatty vegan burgers
- Meat- and poultry-based entrees
- Pizza (vegan versions, too)

Animal-based products

The animal products listed below are high in saturated fat and/or endotoxins. Lean cuts of meat contain less saturated fat than fuller-fat versions.

- Beef
- Butter

- Cheese
- Chicken

- Eggs
- Half-and-half and cream
- Ice cream
- Pork
- Whole milk

Prepackaged foods

Things don't get much better in the bakery and snack aisles. Many prepackaged foods are high in saturated fats and refined sugars and grains, making them pro-inflammatory.

- Candy
- Desserts, breads, and baked goods made with white flour, white sugar, and oils (vegan versions, too)
- Ice cream (vegan versions, too)
- Snack foods made with oil, such as potato chips, tortilla chips, cookies, and crackers
- Sugary drinks, including soda and sports drinks

Homemade desserts

The saturated fats, refined sugars, and refined flours in many homemade desserts can increase inflammation. While making your own cakes, cookies, pies, and puddings results in fresher, tastier, and somewhat healthier foods than store-bought versions, most recipes for homemade sweets include primarily pro-inflammatory ingredients.

Vegetable oils

In addition to dairy butter, certain vegetable oils are high in pro-inflammatory saturated fats.

- Vegan butter
- Vegetable shortening
- Margarine
- Palm oil

The oils listed above are the most pro-inflammatory because of their saturated fat levels, but I avoid all cooking oils in my diet and recipes because of their 100 percent fat content, high calorie count, and potential to harm the inner lining of the arteries, called

The Plant-Based Anti-Inflammatory Cookbook

the endothelium. (For more on this issue, see my post called "What's Wrong with Oil?" on graciousvegan.com.) If you use oil, I recommend olive oil or avocado oil and using as little as possible.

Foods That Reduce Inflammation

And now for the good stuff. A healthy plant-based diet centering on fruits, vegetables, beans, split peas, lentils, whole grains, nuts, and seeds is ideal for reducing inflammation. Foods that are not processed at all are best, but lightly processed plant food like dried fruit, canned beans, hummus, tofu, salsas, and frozen fruits and vegetables are also fine. Recipes like the ones in this cookbook that combine whole or lightly processed plant-based ingredients are also healthy and can help you build filling and satisfying meals.

Replacing tried-and-true meat or cheese dishes you're used to cooking with plant-based recipes can be challenging at first, especially if you cook for a partner or children who may not be as ready to change as you are. As you and they gain experience with a plant-centered diet, though, it will begin to feel more familiar. If you are able to eat healthy plant foods for most of your meals and snacks, you should start to feel better, an added incentive to keep going. If you shift from an animal-based diet to a healthy plant-based diet, it should only take a few weeks before you start to feel the positive effects.

Anti-Inflammatory Superstars

Even within a healthy plant-based diet, there are foods that excel when it comes to lowering chronic inflammation. Researchers continue to work on identifying foods and nutrients that are especially good at bringing down the levels of inflammatory markers in the blood. So far they've found that the following foods are particularly anti-inflammatory.

Ginger and turmeric

These cousins—knobby roots from the same botanical family—are full of antioxidants, some of which are brilliant at neutralizing free radicals (unstable atoms that can cause oxidative stress and inflammation).

Garlic

Garlic contains diallyl disulfide, a compound that limits the effects of pro-inflammatory cytokines.

Green and black tea

Green and black teas contain a type of flavonoid that scavenges unstable oxygen molecules and stops free radicals from forming, decreasing the need for immune cells to be activated.

Foods high in anthocyanins

The antioxidant anthocyanin suppresses pro-inflammatory cytokines and is the source of dark red, purple, blue, and black pigments in fruits, vegetables, legumes, and grains.

Fruits and vegetables

Apples (red, unpeeled)
Berries (blackberries, blueberries, raspberries, strawberries, cranberries, açai, etc.)
Cherries
Eggplants (unpeeled)
Pomegranates
Radishes
Red cabbage
Red onion
Red, purple, and black grapes
Purple asparagus (unpeeled)
Purple cauliflower
Purple kale
Purple sweet potatoes
Purple tomatoes

Legumes
    Black beans
    Kidney beans
    Small red beans

Whole grains
    Black barley
    Black quinoa
    Black rice

Teas
    Hibiscus tea
    Purple tea

Foods high in flavones

Flavones are antioxidants that inhibit certain inflammatory chemical reactions, leading to reduced inflammation and oxidative stress.

- Apples (red, unpeeled)
- Celery
- Chamomile tea
- Citrus (oranges, lemons, limes, etc.)
- Mint
- Parsley
- Red bell peppers
- Rosemary

Foods high in omega-3

Omega-3 fatty acids inhibit production of inflammatory compounds and interrupt several harmful inflammatory processes in our cells.

- Chia seeds
- Flaxseeds
- Hemp seeds
- Pecans
- Walnuts

Cruciferous vegetables

Cruciferous vegetables contain glucosinolates, which can interrupt inflammatory processes, decreasing inflammation and oxidative stress.

- Broccoli
- Brussels sprouts
- Cabbage
- Cauliflower
- Kale
- Spinach

Foods high in fiber

Fiber feeds our beneficial gut bacteria, which in turn release types of short-chain fatty acids that reduce the production of pro-inflammatory proteins.

- Beans, split peas, and lentils
- Fruits and vegetables
- Lima beans, edamame, peas
- Pumpkin seeds, chia seeds, almonds
- Whole grains, including whole wheat spaghetti, barley, oats

As I dug deeper and deeper into harmful pro-inflammatory foods and helpful anti-inflammatory superstars, I increased my own intake of the superstars. I eat berries or a small berry smoothie every morning. I love crisp apples, so I now incorporate the habit of eating a midmorning apple every day. My evening salad's foundation is now baby kale and spinach. And I use a lot of garlic, ginger, and turmeric in my cooking.

Having been lucky to have learned about inflammation and anti-inflammatory eating, I haven't succumbed so far to any of the diseases in my family tree. I'm not on any medications, the numbers on my annual blood test are well within range, and I feel great. The knowledge of specific foods that are pro- and anti-inflammatory has given me extra motivation to eat well. I refuse to have a "body on fire," as some experts refer to chronic inflammation. The only fire I want inside me is the drive to live the healthiest, most productive, connected, and meaningful life I can.

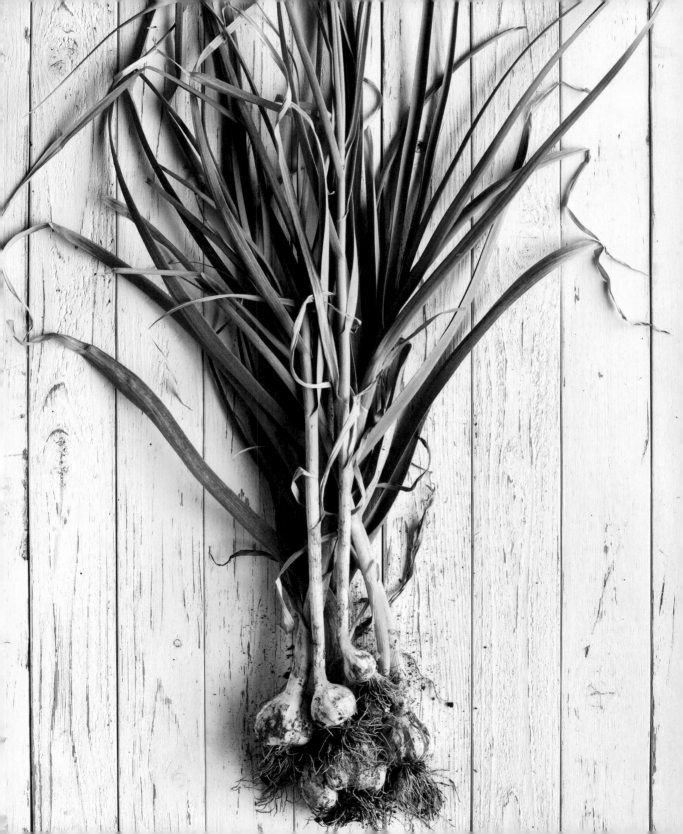

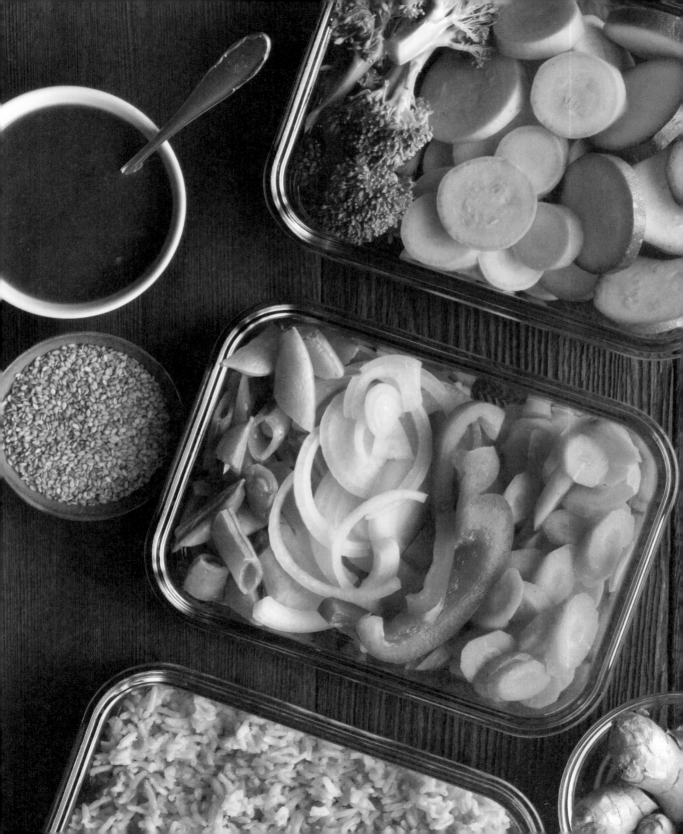

Making Plant-Based Anti-Inflammatory Cooking Work for You

This chapter focuses on the "how" of plant-based cooking so that making anti-inflammatory meals can become familiar and feasible for you. I cover cooking techniques that are important to healthy plant-based cooking, essential equipment, and meal-prep suggestions to help you save valuable time.

Most plant-based cooking steps and skill sets are the same as for more conventional cooking. But new techniques are required to avoid the saturated fats in cooking oils.

Cooking without Oil
Water- or broth-sauté method

Traditional sauté methods use oil. Plant-based anti-inflammatory cooking does not rely on oil, and I, like many cooks, use a water- or broth-sauté method instead.

The water- or broth-sauté method is easiest with nonstick pans, including seasoned cast iron. Pans should be large enough for the vegetable bits to form a single layer, or as close to a single layer as possible, so that the vegetables can brown a bit.

There's no strict right or wrong way to use the water- or broth-sauté method, but if you want as much browning as possible, using less water and adding a little at a time work best. Stirring only occasionally, not constantly, also encourages browning. See instructions below:

Basic water- or broth-sauté method
1. Add the diced vegetables to a skillet or pan and add enough water or broth to form a thin layer on the bottom of the pan. Use a wooden spoon or other utensil to spread out the vegetables.

2. Turn the heat to medium or medium-low. It will take a few minutes for the vegetables to start sizzling.

3. Stir the vegetables every 2 to 3 minutes and spread them out after stirring. If the water evaporates, add more to form a thin layer on the bottom of the pan. You may get some browning on the vegetables or the pan (called "fond"). Use the water and your spoon or spatula to scrub the fond off (or "deglaze") the pan to capture some of the brown in your recipe.

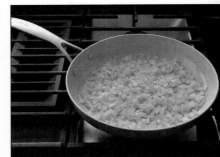

4. Note that mushrooms release their own liquids, so you will likely need less water when sautéing those.

5. If your vegetables include onion, be sure the onion is tender and transparent before continuing with the rest of your recipe. Onions usually take the longest in a vegetable sauté, about 8 to 10 minutes.

Water- or broth-sauté takes a little getting used to, but once you're comfortable with it, it feels very natural. For a video of this technique, see "How to Water Sauté" on my YouTube Channel **Gracious Vegan Kitchen**.

Roasting Vegetables without Oil

Almost every conventional recipe for roasted vegetables calls for oil, sometimes a good amount of it. Oil facilitates high-temperature cooking and the accompanying "Maillard reaction"—the transformation of proteins and sugars into dark brown surfaces with roasted flavor and aroma.

Plant-based recipe developers have come up with a number of ways to roast vegetables without oil.

- Some suggest steaming starchy vegetables before roasting without oil (carrots, potatoes, etc.).
- Others recommend coating vegetables in a little vegetable broth, lemon juice, vinegar, soy sauce, or tamari.

Instead of presteaming or using an acid or broth on the vegetables, I prefer a technique that uses tahini (ground sesame seeds). Tahini is a whole food with natural fat (about half the calories and one-third the fat grams of oil). I replace oil with half-tahini, half-water and add some spices. With high heat in the oven, it's possible to get some of the browning and crispiness of oil roasting with this method without having to presteam the vegetables.

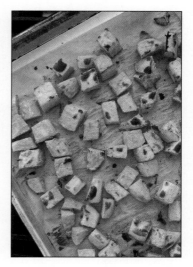

I've found that silicone mats yield less browning, so I either use parchment paper or just put the vegetables directly on a metal sheet pan.

Making Cashew Cream

Cashew cream is a great substitute for half-and-half, heavy cream, or coconut milk. Cashew cream is also one of the easiest nut milks to make, because the cashews dissolve quickly and completely in water, and no straining is required. The key to making good cashew cream is blending long enough to achieve an absolutely smooth texture. Soaking the raw cashews first facilitates this silkiness. High-speed blenders are able to break down unsoaked cashews, but I still soak the nuts if my schedule allows.

Cashew cream

1. Soak raw cashews for at least 2 hours in cold or room temperature water, or pour boiling water over them, cover them, and let them stand for 20 minutes. In either case, drain before using.
2. It's especially important to presoak the cashews if you want to use a small (a.k.a. bullet or personal) or regular blender. Blending times will be longer with these types of blenders compared with high-speed models. But they do work. This is not a job for the food processor, which doesn't do well with so much liquid.
3. If the recipe calls for more than twice the amount of water as cashews, I recommend that you start by blending the cashews first with a portion of the water—just to cover the cashews in the blender. Blend to a smooth consistency,

then add the remaining water and blend. This ensures that the cashew cream will be as smooth as possible without grit.

4. To make cashew milk for drinking and using in oatmeal or cereal, soak and drain ⅔ cup raw cashews, then blend them first with 1 cup water, then add 2 more cups water. I recommend adding 1–2 teaspoons vanilla extract, 1 large pinch cinnamon, and maple syrup to taste.

Baking Burgers

Most veggie burger recipes call for panfrying the burgers before serving. The good news is that healthy veggie burgers can be baked without oil and still come out fully cooked—not mushy—with brown, crispy edges.

In my burger recipes I recommend using relatively high heat in the oven (400°F or 425°F) and lining the pan with parchment paper or a silicone mat. After baking about 15 minutes on one side, flip the burgers over and bake them for 10 to 15 minutes more. As long as the recipe has the right ingredients for holding the burgers together without too much squishiness, the baked burgers will have an excellent texture.

Air-Frying Foods That Are Usually Fried

Air frying is a great way to cook foods without having to use oil. Perhaps the best-known air-fried dish is French fries without oil. Simply cut the potatoes into sticks or wedges, toss them with some seasonings (I like smoked paprika, nutritional yeast, and salt), and air fry for 20 to 22 minutes (or more) at 400°F, tossing the fries at least once during cooking time to redistribute them in the basket. The fries taste yummy, with many fewer calories and grams of fat than their deep-fried cousins.

The same air-fry technique can be used with other vegetables. Wedges or cubes of vegetables can be coated with seasoning, vinegar, a tahini mixture, or other light sauce. The air fryer produces fantastic baked potatoes as well, crispy on the outside and fluffy on the inside.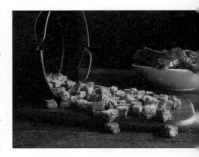

Other recipes work well in the air fryer without oil. I air fry taquitos, falafel, tofu cubes, croutons, and roasted chickpeas, among others. The air fryer cooks food more quickly than the oven, doesn't require long preheating times, and doesn't turn the kitchen into a sauna.

Steaming Vegetables in a Pressure Cooker

A pressure cooker makes cooking batches of vegetables easier and more enjoyable for a few reasons:

- Faster cooking times
- Fewer dishes and pots to clean
- Hands-off cooking, so you can do other things while the vegetables cook
- Less nutrient loss than boiling vegetables on the stove

I cook the following vegetables in my electric pressure cooker using a "zero-minute" steaming method (see below). Sometimes I mix and cook them together, but I usually cook them separately.

- Broccoli
- Brussels sprouts
- Cauliflower
- Dark leafy greens (kale, collard greens, mustard greens)
- Green beans

"Zero-Minute" Steaming Method

1. Prep the vegetables (i.e., trim and cut them into chunks, florets, etc.).
2. Rinse the vegetables (you can use the steamer basket for this).
3. Set up the pressure cooker: use the included steamer basket or a conventional steamer basket. Having handles helps when you take them out after cooking.
4. Pour 1 to 1½ cups of water into the pressure cooker.
5. Pile the vegetables into the basket and lock the lid.
6. Turn the knob to "Sealing," use the "Steam" mode, and lower the minutes to 0 (zero).

7. When pressure is reached and the pressure cooker signals "done," immediately move the knob to "Venting." (I use a spoon to move it, since the steam and the lid are really hot.)

8. Once the steam is released and the tiny pressure valve drops (this takes 1 to 3 minutes), remove the lid and lift out the vegetables (I use oven mitts).

I use the same method for the following vegetables, but they need more minutes on "Steam."

- Butternut squash, sliced—3 minutes
- Carrots, sliced—2 minutes
- Spaghetti squash, halved—6 minutes
- Sweet potatoes and white/yellow potatoes, cubed—2 to 3 minutes (firmer vs. softer)

You can adjust these timings to your taste once you get the hang of this method.

I don't cook the following vegetables in my pressure cooker because they are too delicate for the high-pressure blast, in my opinion, but I encourage you to find other opinions online and decide for yourself.

- Asparagus
- Cabbage
- Corn
- Eggplant
- Frozen vegetables
- Peas
- Spinach
- Swiss chard

Helpful Equipment for Plant-Based Cooking
Blenders

I use at least one of my blenders every day. They're indispensable for plant-based cooking. Blenders give the following types of mixtures a perfect silky-smooth texture that no other appliance can match.

- Cashew cream
- Creamy or pureed soups
- Homemade nondairy milk
- Plant-based cheeses

- Plant-based mayonnaise
- Salad dressings
- Sauces

I have three blenders and use them for different purposes.

- **High-speed blender**: This blender is the most powerful and creates the silkiest texture. It can handle large mixtures, even whole recipes of soups. The only limitation is that it doesn't blend small recipes well (under 2 cups). It needs a critical mass to create the vortex that allows the blades to break everything down.
- **Small/bullet/personal blender**: This smaller blender isn't as powerful as a high-speed blender, but it's perfect for smoothies and small batches of cashew cream, salad dressings, and sauces. It can also grind dry chia seeds and spices.
- **Stick/immersion blender**: This blender is the least powerful of the three, but it's handy and safe for pureeing soups or sauces right in their cooking pans.

Food processor

As opposed to a blender, a food processor works best with dry or semidry mixtures, which blenders are not able to handle. The food processor has a flat blade that sits at the bottom of its flat bowl, and with every turn, the blade cuts through whatever is sitting on the bottom of the bowl.

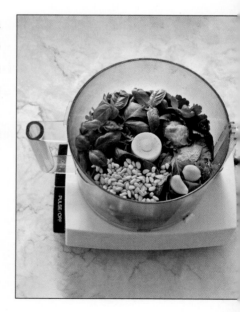

The food processor is great at the following types of tasks:

- Blending pesto
- Chopping fresh herbs
- Chopping nuts
- Creating chunky veggie burger and falafel mixtures
- Creating no-bake cookies and pie crusts
- Making bean dips
- Turning nuts into plant-based Parmesan cheese and other dry "cheeses"

Making Plant-Based Anti-Inflammatory Cooking Work for You

I recommend a 10- or 11-cup food processor, but the 8-cup size or smaller also works well if you don't need to make large batches of food.

Nonstick skillets

Nonstick skillets are essential tools for anti-inflammatory recipes because oil is not used in healthy plant-based cooking. With good nonstick skillets, you can sauté vegetables in water or broth, make stir-fries, and cook scrambled tofu and other foods without the use of oil.

There are several types of nonstick coatings, but ceramic nonstick coatings are considered the best, and this has proven true in my kitchen. There are many excellent brands with a variety of sizes, prices, and metal composition. I use my 10-inch and 8-inch skillets the most, but I also have a 12-inch skillet for larger jobs. Be careful that the pan you buy isn't too heavy to lift easily with one arm (when you're scooping hot food out of the skillet).

If you take care of your ceramic nonstick skillets—by avoiding metal utensils, washing by hand (without metal scouring pads), and not piling other pans on top of them without a soft divider—they will last many years.

Tips, Tricks, and Other Efficiencies for Plant-Based Cooking

If you cook for the household, even if it's a household of one, it means putting a lot of meals on the table day in, day out. I hope the techniques below make cooking anti-inflammatory meals easier for you.

Freezing

Even if you don't have an extra freezer, you can make your cooking go further with a well-tended freezer. The key is to even out the "deposits" and "withdrawals" to maintain a good balance. You can freeze whole meals or individual components depending on your preference.

I try to make enough of most dishes I cook to eat two times during the week with enough left over to freeze for at least one meal in the future. My "steady state" is to cook three new dinners a week with the extra night coming from the freezer. Sometimes I get away with two new dinners a week. I prefer not to cook every night, so using the freezer in this way works for me.

Plant-based freezer meals

Here's a list of plant-based dishes that you can make to completion, then freeze. I recommend freezing dishes in individual portion sizes for easier thawing and reheating. Even though I'm a passionate cook, I love seeing complete meals in the freezer, knowing I'll get the night off from cooking.

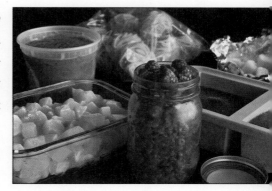

- Chili
- Eggplant parmigiana
- Enchiladas or enchilada casserole
- Energy bites and healthy cookies
- Falafel balls
- Healthy cakes
- Lasagna and other baked pasta dishes
- Scalloped corn
- Shepherd's pie
- Most curries (except potato-heavy curries)
- Most soups and stews (except those that are heavy on potatoes or rice)
- Pizza and calzones (although they never come out quite like freshly baked)
- Sloppy Joe filling
- Steel-cut oatmeal and other cooked whole grain hot cereals
- Vegan meat-like crumbles
- Vegan meatballs
- Veggie burgers

Making Plant-Based Anti-Inflammatory Cooking Work for You

Plant-based freezer meal components

If mix and match is more your style or you like to make extra of certain components that you use a lot, here's a list of items that freeze well. The good news is that most plant-based components freeze well!

- Avocado puree and guacamole
- Cooked grains (quinoa, millet, etc.)
- Cooked legumes (lentils, beans, chickpeas, refried beans)
- Cooked vegetables (greens, broccoli, cauliflower, beets, carrots, summer and winter squash, sweet potatoes, mashed potatoes; note that roasted vegetables will lose their crispness if you freeze them)
- Fresh herbs (note that some herbs retain their texture, like bay leaves, curry leaves, and kaffir lime leaves, but most herbs—like basil, cilantro, and parsley—lose their texture but can be used in recipes like soups, casseroles, and sauces)
- Leftover ingredients like tomato paste, tomato sauce, curry paste, and aquafaba
- Plant-based cheeses and dairy (Parmesan, ricotta, crema, sour cream, cashew cream, "goat" cheese, etc.)
- Raw garlic, chopped
- Raw onion, chopped
- Ripe or overripe bananas (great for smoothies and nice cream; I slice them before freezing)
- Sauces (tomato-based sauces like marinara, pizza, enchilada; nut- and seed-based sauces like tahini sauce, peanut sauce, and cashew-based cream sauces; gravies; pesto of all kinds; curry sauces)
- Whole grain cooked pasta

It's important to label your items unless their identity is crystal clear. I use masking tape and a permanent marker. You can date the item if you are concerned you won't use it within 3 to 4 months.

Foods that don't freeze well

- Avocado, whole or sliced (note that guacamole and avocado puree with a little lemon juice freeze well)
- Cooked asparagus comes out very wilted if frozen
- Cooked pasta tossed with a sauce comes out dry, soggy, and swollen when frozen
- Cooked potato chunks usually turn grainy when frozen (note that mashed potatoes freeze well)
- Fully cooked rice can turn mealy when frozen (best results come when you don't overcook the rice and you use frozen rice within a month or so)

Freezer storage options

Here's a list of safe containers for freezing complete meals or components:

- Heavy-duty foil (you can wrap the food in parchment paper first if you don't want foil touching your food)
- Freezer-safe glass dishes with snap-on lids
- Mason jars (wide-mouth are easiest)
- Plastic containers (BPA-free)
- Plastic freezer bags (BPA-free)
- Silicone storage bags
- Soup "cubes" that freeze 1- or 2-cup portions
- Vacuum sealed packages

Meal Prep

Although every cook has their own unique style of meal prep, there are essentially two types:

- Batch cooking
- Ingredient prep

Or maybe "no prep" is your style—maybe you cook a dish from start to finish right before eating it. That's perfectly okay if you have the time to do so.

Batch cooking is making one or more dishes ahead of time and storing the completed dishes in the refrigerator or freezer. This usually requires setting aside a chunk of time at least once a week, the rule of thumb being three hours. Some people batch cook on Sunday before the work and school weeks begin. Some don't have a set day but figure out a half-day each week when they will batch cook. Batch cooking doesn't work well for dishes that need to be cooked right before eating, such as stir-fries, tacos, pasta tossed with sauce, or salads that call for lettuce or greens to be tossed with a dressing.

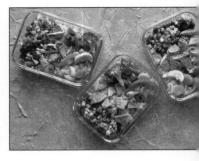

Ingredient prep is making the components of a dish beforehand, then putting them together and cooking them right before eating. This is the kind of prep I tend to do—it just seems to go with my personality and schedule. You can ingredient prep once a week—similar to batch cooking but without completing the dishes—or you can ingredient prep the day of the meal when you get little pockets of time free.

Whether you meal prep during your weekly Zoom call with your sister on Sunday afternoon or in snatches of time while working at home, anything you do ahead of time relieves pressure at the dinner hour. It may take a little while to form the habit if you don't already prep, but once you do, I predict you'll love the feeling of not having to start cooking at square one when your stomach is rumbling and it's time to get dinner on the table.

Semi-homemade

Although healthy anti-inflammatory cooking avoids processed foods, there are still whole-food items you can buy in supermarkets to make meal preparation easier. Some people might say they don't want to pay for something they can do themselves—like peel and cube a butternut squash. Others would say the money is worth the time savings. To each their own.

Vegetables: There are many shortcuts if you don't want to trim, clean, and chop vegetables yourself.

- Bags and clamshells of fresh greens and lettuce
- Bags or containers of cabbage slaw and broccoli slaw
- Bags or containers of fresh prechopped vegetables (e.g., onions, carrots, celery)
- Canned vegetables
- Containers of precubed butternut squash and sliced mushrooms
- Frozen cauliflower rice
- Frozen spiralized vegetables
- Frozen vegetables and vegetable medleys
- Precut vegetable sticks

Some cooks have strong opinions about the texture and/or taste of canned or frozen vegetables, but if you and your family like them, go for it. Some people worry about lost vitamins, minerals, and micronutrients. There are so many variables contributing to loss of nutrients—time from harvest to freezing or eating, type of vegetable, cooking method, etc.—that it's almost impossible to make decisions based on lost nutrients. I say, eat lots of vegetables, whether frozen, canned, prechopped, bagged, home prepped, direct from the field, organic, or not organic. They all contain fiber, water, minerals, and some amount of their original vitamins and micronutrients.

Legumes: Legumes don't have to be cooked from a dry state to get the nutritional whole-food benefits. Many of us use canned beans, and low-sodium beans are an excellent semi-homemade solution in recipes. Some stores like Trader Joe's also feature refrigerated steamed legumes. Here are the main choices of prepared whole-food legumes:

- Canned beans and lentils (low sodium is best; draining and rinsing beans also decreases the sodium content)
- Canned chili beans
- Canned refried beans (no fat)
- Frozen black-eyed peas
- Frozen lima beans, green peas, and edamame (all are technically legumes)
- Presteamed lentils

Making Plant-Based Anti-Inflammatory Cooking Work for You

Whole grains: Whole grains are another critical part of healthy plant-based cooking, and a few shortcuts are available. For these and all products, it's important to read the label to make sure there are no animal or processed ingredients lurking inside.

- Brown rice and other grain mixes (dry)
- Frozen cooked brown rice
- Shelf-stable packets of cooked whole grains and brown rice

See the boxed text here for shortcut products to approach with caution. It's important to read labels to find out what's really in there.

Read labels carefully

Make sure you know what's in these shortcut items before you buy:

- Salad kits (usually contain oil in the dressing)
- Plant-based bowls (usually contain oil)
- Vegan or plant-based dips and sauces (usually contain oil and processed ingredients)
- Veggie burgers (usually contain oil and processed ingredients)

Conclusion

Cooking is an art, a science, a hobby, a job, a chore, a pleasure, an act of love, an opportunity to meditate, a hurried race against the clock—sometimes all of these at once. We are all at different stages and circumstances in our kitchen, each of us bringing a unique set of experiences, memories, and skillsets. But we are part of a human activity that's been around for tens of thousands of years. By necessity we create a style of cooking that is distinctively ours. With these tips for efficient and healthy anti-inflammatory cooking, I hope I've provided some ways for you to more easily and quickly reach your goals for decreasing chronic inflammation.

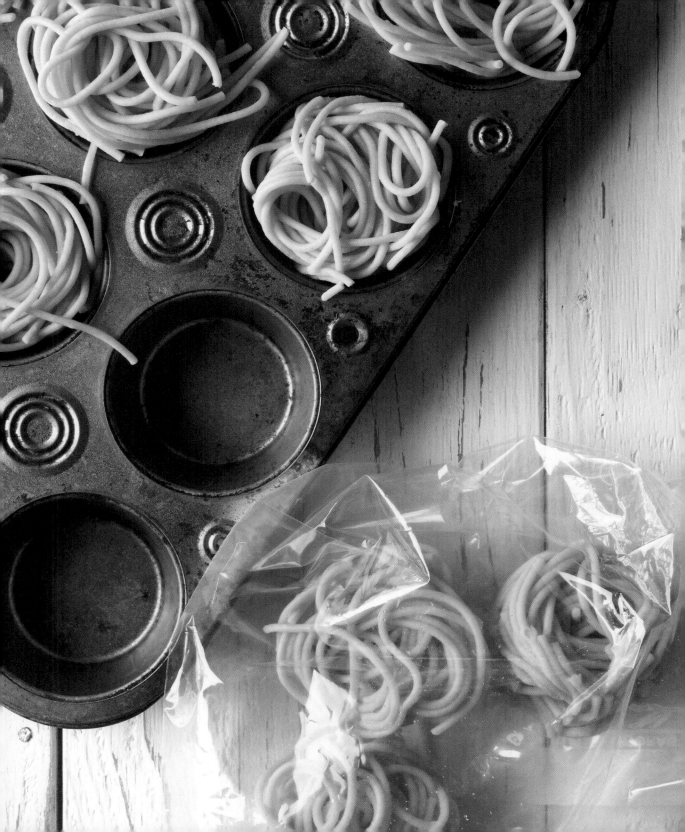

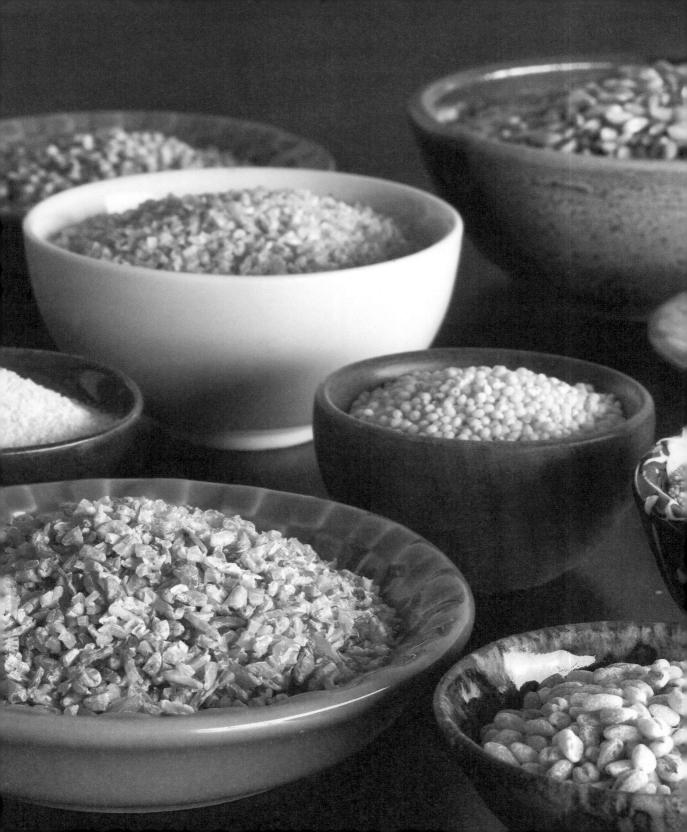

Whole Grains Cooking Guide

Stovetop Directions

Rinse the grains if you wish. (I recommend it for rice, at least.) Bring the liquid to a boil in a saucepan, stir in the grains, and bring the mixture back to a boil. It's optional to add salt as well: I recommend ⅛–¼ teaspoon per cup of uncooked grains. Then, reduce the heat to low, cover the pot, and simmer gently until the grains are tender. Use the following chart as a guide and taste the grains to see if they need more time or liquid. When the grains reach the desired texture, remove the pot from the stove and fluff the grains with a fork. Let the grains cool with the lid slightly ajar for 5 to 10 minutes, then pour off any liquid that remains.

Electric Pressure Cooker (Such as an Instant Pot®) Instructions

Rinse the grains if you wish. (I recommend it for rice, at least.) Add the liquid and grains to the pressure cooker pot. It's optional to add salt as well: I recommend ⅛–¼ teaspoon per cup of uncooked grains. Next, lock the lid, turn the knob to "Sealing," use the "High," "Pressure Cook," "Multigrain," or "Manual" mode, and set for the recommended number of minutes.

Wait for 10 minutes after the pressure cooker is done, then move the knob to "Venting" and release the remaining steam before opening the lid. Check if the grains are done. If they are done, fluff the grains with a fork and allow them to sit for about 5 minutes before serving. If they are not done, add about ¼ cup water, if needed, bring the cooker back up to pressure, and cook the grains for 1 minute or 2 longer.

These amounts are for 1 cup uncooked grains but they can be doubled or tripled accordingly. The cooking times on the stove or in the pressure cooker can stay the same when doubled or tripled.

Uncooked grain (1 cup)	Simmering duration on the stovetop	Water or vegetable broth	Duration at high pressure	Water or vegetable broth
Barley, pearled	45 to 60 minutes	3 cups	20 minutes	2 cups
Buckwheat groats	20 to 25 minutes	2 cups	5 minutes	1½ cups
Farro, pearled	15 to 20 minutes	2½ cups	8 minutes	1½ cups
Freekeh	20 to 25 minutes	2½ cups	10 minutes	1⅔ cups
Millet	25 to 30 minutes	2½ cups	11 minutes	1⅓ cups
Oats, steel-cut	30 to 35 minutes	4 cups	5 minutes	3½ cups
Quinoa, red or white	12 to 15 minutes	2 cups	2 minutes for white, 3 minutes for red	1¼ cups
Rice, black	40 to 50 minutes	2 cups	18 minutes	1⅛ cups
Rice, brown	40 to 50 minutes	2½ cups	22 minutes	1⅓ cups
Rice, wild	40 to 60 minutes	3 cups	23 minutes	1⅓ cups
Sorghum	25 to 40 minutes	4 cups	23 minutes	2½ cups
Spelt	65 to 80 minutes (40 to 60 minutes if presoaked)	3 cups	25 minutes	1½ cups
Wheat berries	60 to 90 minutes (40 to 60 minutes if presoaked)	4 cups	30 minutes	3 cups

The Plant-Based Anti-Inflammatory Cookbook

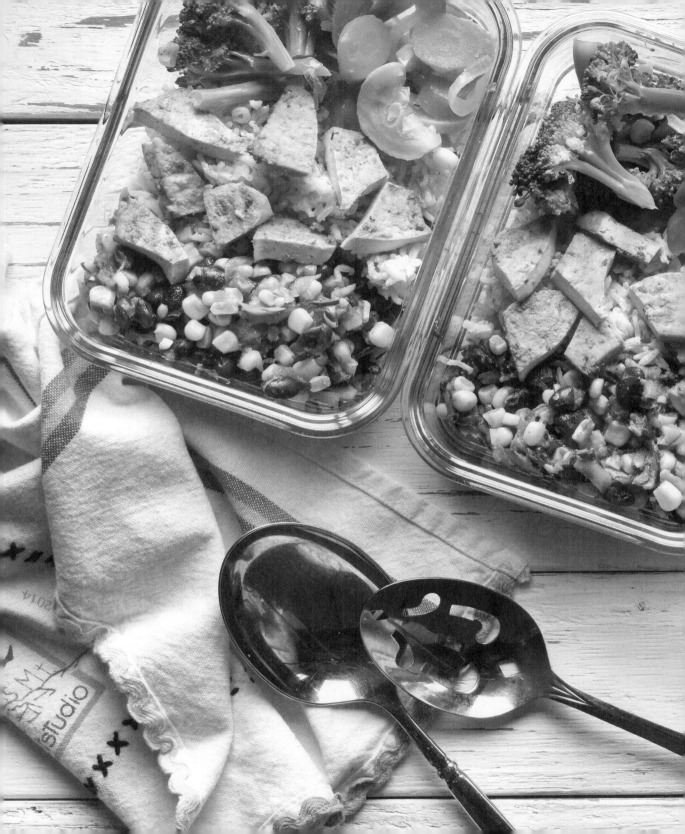

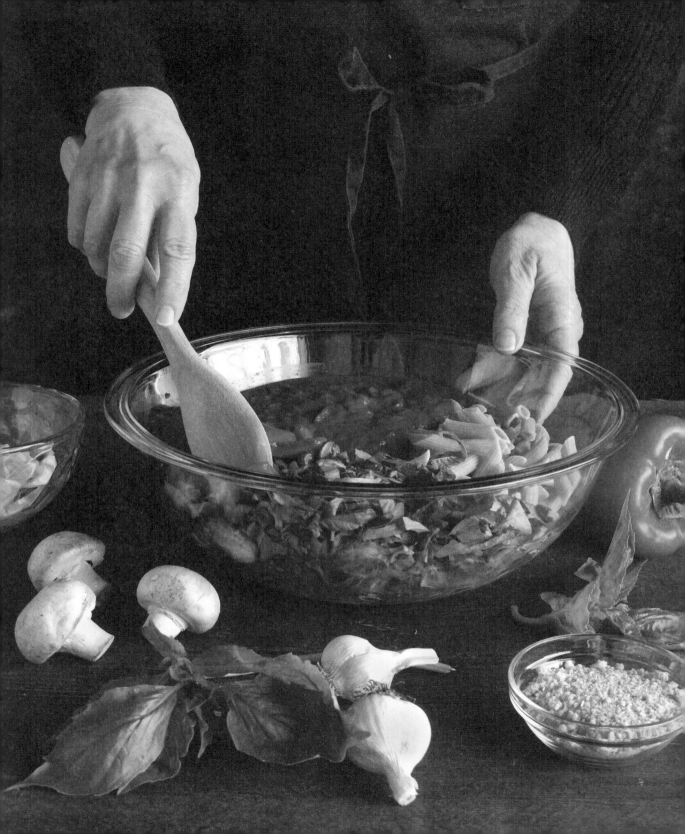

PART II
Recipes

Recipe Format

My recipes may look a little unconventional at first. I use the "action method" format, which means that the ingredients are interpolated within the instructions rather than listed up front. Other cookbooks that use this method include *The Joy of Cooking*, originally by Irma Rombacher, and *The Art of Simple Food* by Alice Waters.

This method is helpful when prepping ingredients for a dish. You can see immediately which ingredients are used in each step of the recipe, and you can prep and store the ingredients together in advance.

I hope you find this format as efficient as I do, once you get used to it. To use this format, simply complete each step with the ingredients listed directly under that step, then move to the next step.

Anti-Inflammatory Superstars

The anti-inflammatory superstars in each recipe are **green**. I hope this helps you as you make choices about ingredients and substitutions.

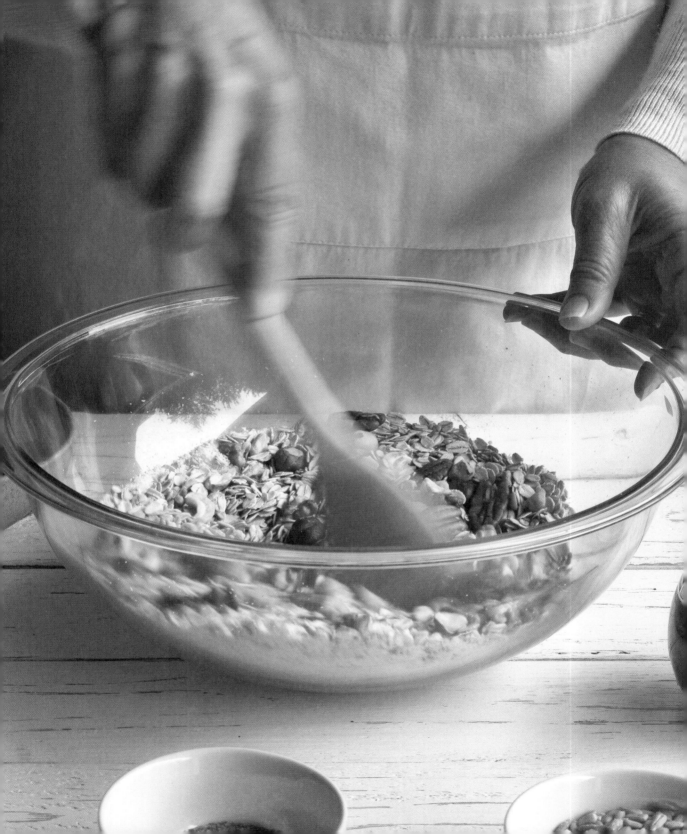

Breakfast, Brunch, and Beverages

We're all so different about breakfast. Some people skip it entirely. Some go for a smoothie and energy bar. Some have eaten eggs for breakfast most of their lives and want tasty, filling alternatives for a plant-based lifestyle.

In this chapter, I start with savory options for those who miss eggs. Then, I move to fruit and cereal, including hot cereals. Finally, I offer several nutrient-dense smoothies and teas. There's something for everyone here—whether for a quick weekday anti-inflammatory boost or a more leisurely weekend spread.

The possibilities for eating and drinking anti-inflammatory superstars at breakfast are many. Berries and cherries shine in parfaits and smoothies. Red bell peppers are natural in scrambles, with potatoes, and on toast. Oranges and lemons flavor teas, smoothies, and even granola. Steel-cut oats provide highly beneficial fiber. Breakfast can start your day with an anti-inflammatory advantage.

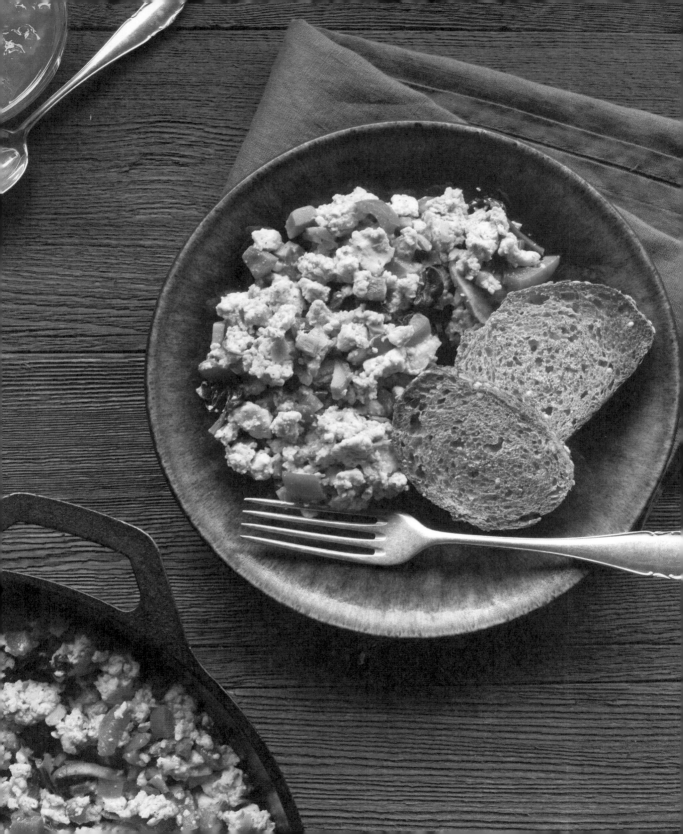

Brunch-Worthy Vegetable Scramble

Makes 4 servings

What makes this scramble brunch-worthy is the creaminess created by blending a few raw cashews with tofu and nondairy milk. It cozies up well next to Roasted Breakfast Potatoes (page 56) and whole grain toast. You can substitute the mushrooms and bell peppers with any vegetables you have on hand. It's worth seeking out kala namak (see box) for a better "eggy" taste. Any leftovers would make a great topping for toast later in the week.

Soak the cashews. Soak the cashews in water for 2 hours or pour boiling water over them, cover, let them soak for about 20 minutes, and drain them. Set aside.

2 tablespoons raw cashews

Start the scramble. Water sauté the following ingredients in a large skillet until the onions are tender and transparent and the liquid released by the mushrooms is fully evaporated, 8 to 10 minutes.

¼ cup diced onion (red, yellow, or white)
1 cup diced or sliced cremini or white button mushrooms (about 4 mushrooms)
½ cup diced red bell pepper

Prep the tofu. In the meantime, drain the tofu and press a kitchen towel or paper towels onto all sides of the tofu to reduce the excess liquid.

16 ounces firm tofu

Take about ⅔ of the tofu and crumble it into chunks about the size of raspberries. Set the chunks aside. Add the remaining tofu to a small blender and blend it until smooth with the following ingredients.

The soaked and drained cashews
½ cup unsweetened nondairy milk
1½ teaspoons nutritional yeast
1 teaspoon kala namak
¾ teaspoon turmeric
Freshly ground black pepper to taste

Finish the scramble. When the water sauté is complete, add the following ingredients to the skillet and cook on medium-low heat for 3 to 7 minutes, scraping across the bottom of the pan every minute or so (since cashews can burn), until it reaches your desired consistency (wetter or drier).

The crumbled tofu

The blended tofu mixture

1 packed cup baby spinach

¾ teaspoon thyme

¾ teaspoon oregano

¼ teaspoon garlic powder

Taste for seasonings and adjust. The scramble is ready to serve. The scramble will keep in the refrigerator for a few days. It does not freeze well.

Kala namak

Kala namak is a type of salt with high sulfur content harvested from volcanic mines. This means it's perfect for plant-based dishes that benefit from an eggy taste and smell. It's also called Himalayan black salt, Indian black salt, or just black salt. Its color is more often pink or gray rather than black, despite the name. Kala namak is great in tofu scrambles like this one and also plant-based mayo, Eggless Egg Salad (page 104), or any dish that would benefit from an egg-like taste and smell.

Hummus Toast and Variations

Makes as many servings as you desire

If you are looking to ditch eggs in the morning, I recommend hummus toast. A quarter cup of hummus offers three to four times more protein than half an avocado, and the variations on hummus toast are at least as numerous as avocado toast. My personal favorite is "Hiker's Special"—created by my sister and me for sandwiches when we go on long day-hikes.

Hummus toast starts, of course, with spreading hummus on 1 or 2 pieces of toast.

Whole grain bread is healthiest for the toast (thick and thin slices both work well)
Homemade or store-bought hummus in various flavors such as red pepper, garlic, or black bean (if using store-bought, look for hummus that has no added oil)

Here are five fun combinations for toppings:

Greek salad

Halved Kalamata olives, capers, diced tomatoes, diced red onion, diced cucumbers, a sprinkling of dried oregano, and a splash of red wine vinegar

Margarita

Sliced tomatoes, fresh basil leaves, salt, pepper, and a generous splash of balsamic vinegar

Pico de gallo

Diced tomatoes, diced red onion, cilantro, sliced jalapeños, and a generous splash of lime juice

Hiker's Special

Homemade or store-bought roasted red bell peppers (drained, rinsed, and patted dry), walnut pieces, and halved Kalamata or California olives

Tzatziki

Cucumber ribbons dotted with vegan (unsweetened) yogurt mixed with salt and garlic powder

You can also make up your own combination from any of these topping ideas:

Vegetables
Any roasted vegetable
Raw or roasted bell peppers

Thinly sliced celery
Sliced, ribboned, or diced cucumbers
Grated beets

(Continued on page 55)

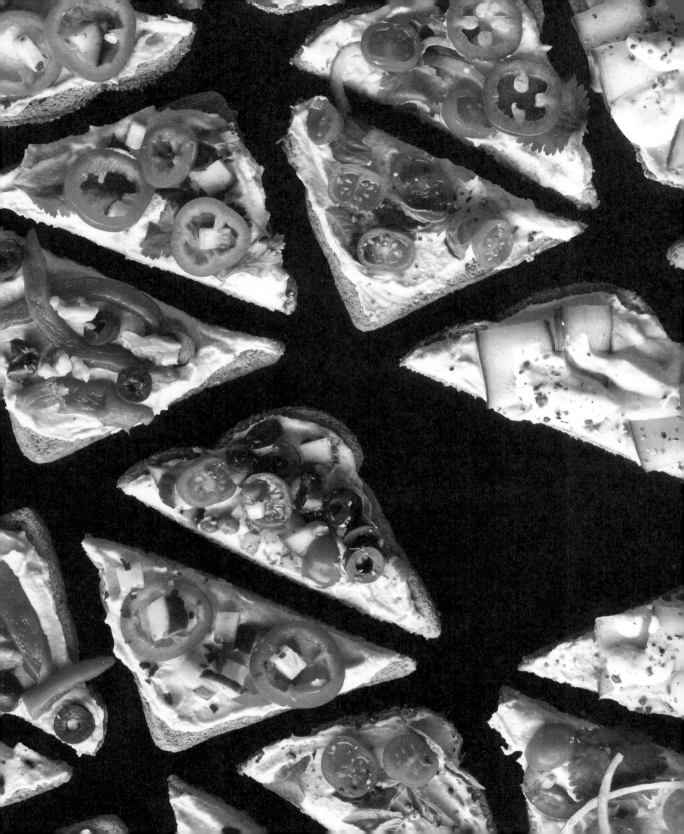

Grated carrots
Jalapeños or other chiles
Onions (red, yellow, white, or pickled)
Sliced radishes
Sundried tomatoes
Thinly shredded cabbage
Tomatoes

Spice mixes

Dukkah
Za'atar
Everything but the Bagel seasoning
Spike seasoning

Other

Cilantro
Parsley
Raw spinach leaves
Salad greens
Kalamata olives
California olives
Roasted nuts and seeds
Pesto
Tapenade

Splashes

Any kind of vinegar or flavored vinegar
Lime or lemon juice

Spice mixes

It's impossible to overstate the effect of vibrant spice mixes on dishes like hummus and avocado toast. I've become particularly attached to dukkah, a heady blend of nuts, seeds, and spices originally from Egypt, as well as za'atar, with historical roots throughout the Middle East and northern Africa, with a sharper taste from sumac, but also the more familiar oregano, thyme, and sesame seeds. (See graciousvegan.com for these spice mix recipes, or you can buy them already made.) You may have other favorite mixes—sprinkle away! The lower the salt, the better. Find your favorite and liven up your toast, cooked or roasted vegetables, pasta, grains, soups, and baked potatoes. As a bonus, spices are full of antioxidants.

Roasted Breakfast Potatoes

Makes 4 servings

Most recipes for breakfast potatoes and hash browns call for several tablespoons of oil. Here I use a little soy sauce and tahini with spices to coat the potatoes, and this results in lovely cubes that are soft on the inside and crisp on the outside. These potatoes complement the Brunch-Worthy Vegetable Scramble (page 51) for a special breakfast, but, really, these potatoes would be great for dinner, too. Adding salsa or a plant-based cheese sauce (see graciousvegan.com for recipes) would take these potatoes to another level!

Preheat the oven to 425°F. Line a sheet pan with parchment paper or a silicone mat. Add the following ingredients to a large bowl and toss them well with a spatula to coat all the potato chunks.

> **1 pound russet, Yukon, or red potatoes, cut into ½"–¾" chunks (no need to peel the potatoes)**
>
> **2 teaspoons soy sauce or tamari**
>
> **2 teaspoons tahini**
>
> **1 teaspoon water**
>
> **½ teaspoon thyme**
>
> **½ teaspoon paprika**
>
> **½ teaspoon smoked paprika**
>
> **⅛ teaspoon garlic powder**
>
> **Freshly ground black pepper to taste**

Spread the mixture out on the sheet pan. Roast for 10 minutes, then take the pan out of the oven, flip the potatoes, add the following ingredients, and distribute everything evenly across the pan.

> **½ medium red, yellow, or white onion, diced (about ¾ cup)**
>
> **¾ cup diced red bell pepper**

Roast for another 10 to 15 minutes and check for tenderness. If the potatoes are not tender, roast for another 5 minutes and test again. Once they are well roasted, they are ready to serve. They will keep for about a week in the refrigerator. They do not freeze well.

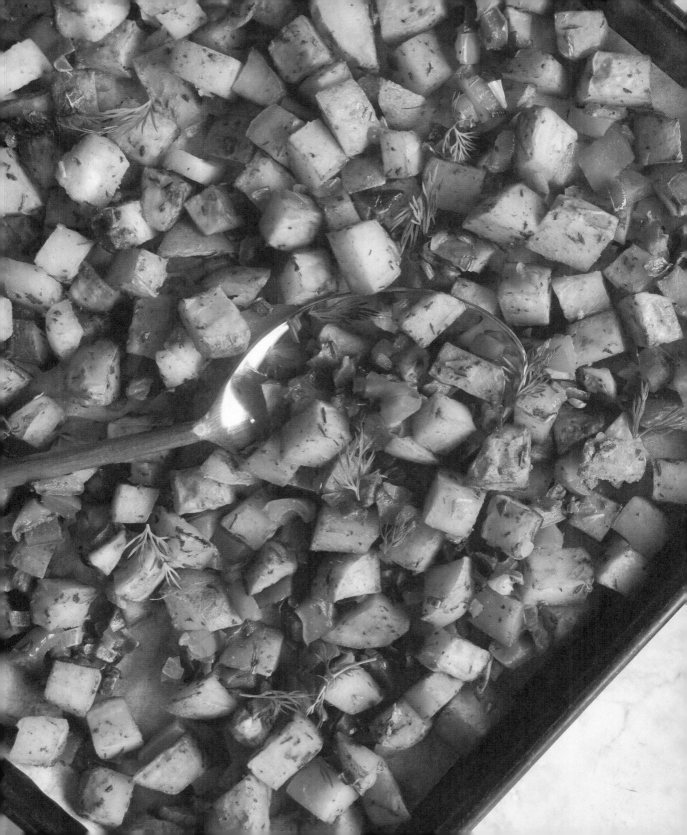

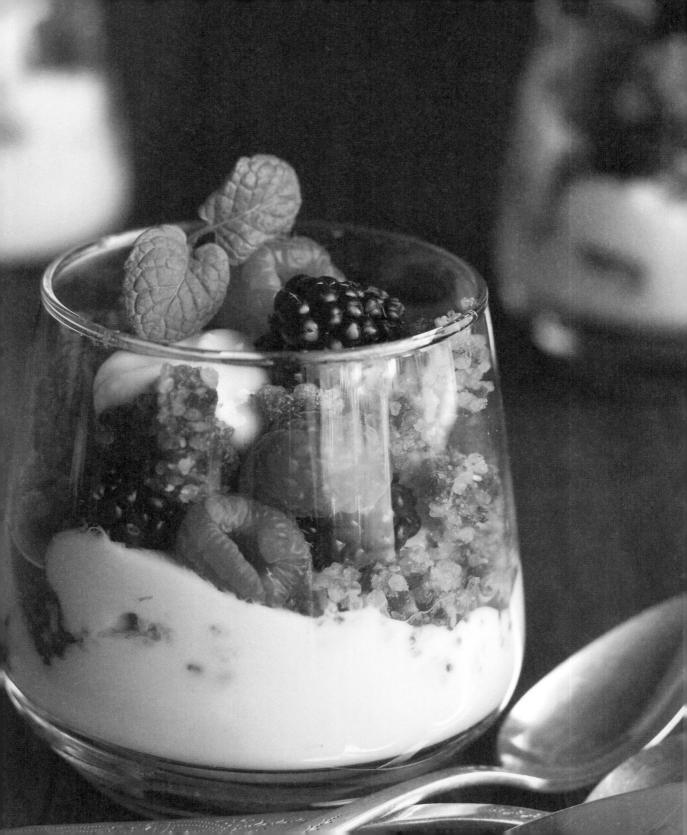

Berry, Yogurt, and Soft Crumble Parfaits

Makes 4 servings

One day I suddenly realized that the grainy layer in a breakfast fruit parfait didn't have to be dry and crunchy. I could use cooked grains in it! Thus was born the "soft crumble" in this recipe. I love that the parfait holds its shape even 24 or 48 hours after layering the parfaits. The fruit you use can reflect what's in season—berries in spring, cherries in early summer, peaches and melons in late summer, and cooked apples and pears in fall.

Make the crumble. Add the following ingredients to a food processor and process until the date pieces are very small and there is still good texture in the crumble, about 30 seconds.

8 pitted Medjool dates, each cut into 2–3 pieces
¾ cup cooked quinoa*
¼ cup nuts or seeds, raw or roasted
½ tablespoon chia seeds
½ tablespoon flaxseed meal
½ teaspoon cinnamon
Dash of vanilla powder or splash of vanilla extract

Assemble the parfaits. Spoon a layer of yogurt into 4 individual bowls or parfait glasses.

2 cups nondairy yogurt**

Add a layer of berries, then sprinkle with a layer of the crumble. Repeat the layering once or twice more, depending on the height of the bowl or glass, ending with a layer of crumble.

2–3 cups berries such as blueberries, strawberries, raspberries, and/or blackberries—washed, dried, and sliced as desired

The parfaits are ready to serve or will stay fresh in the refrigerator for 24 to 48 hours. The parfaits do not freeze well.

---

* You can substitute with cooked brown rice, millet, or other cooked grain, but if you do, I recommend making the homemade crumble topping right before serving, since some cooked grains can get hard if stored for hours in the refrigerator.

** I prefer unsweetened plant-based yogurt, but any favorite will do. See graciousvegan.com for how to make soy milk yogurt in an electric pressure cooker. I recommend straining homemade yogurt to make it thicker for this recipe.

Orange-Spice Granola

Makes 7½ cups

The genius ingredient in this granola is date syrup. The syrup sweetens and combines with chia seeds and flaxseed meal to create wonderful crunchy clusters. The date syrup also substitutes, along with almond butter, for oil. You can customize the types of nuts and dried fruit. My favorite way to eat this granola is with berries and homemade soy yogurt. I also top my regular Daily Habit Berry Smoothie Bowl (page 71) with it. The granola tastes great with nondairy milk in a bowl, on toast with nut butter, in fruit parfaits, and by itself as a snack. This granola is hard to resist!

Preheat the oven to 300°F. Line 2 baking sheets with parchment paper or silicone mats.

Stir together the following dry ingredients in a large bowl.

> **2 cups old fashioned oats**
> **1⅓ cups roughly chopped nuts (all one kind or a combination of walnuts, almonds, hazelnuts, cashews, pecans, Brazil nuts, etc.)**
> **⅓ cup unsweetened shredded coconut or larger unsweetened coconut flakes**
> **¼ cup raw seeds (sunflower, pumpkin, sesame, hemp, etc.)**
> **1½ tablespoons chia seeds**
> **1½ tablespoons flaxseed meal**
> **Zest from 1 orange**
> **½ teaspoon nutmeg**
> **⅛– ¼ teaspoon salt (optional)**

In a separate bowl, whisk together the following wet ingredients.

> **½ cup date syrup or ⅔ cup maple syrup**
> **2 tablespoons almond butter**
> **1 tablespoon water**
> **2 teaspoons vanilla extract or vanilla powder**

Pour the wet ingredients into the dry ingredients. Stir all the ingredients together so that they are well combined and coated. Divide the mixture between the 2 pans and spread it into a thin, even layer on the parchment or mats.

Bake the granola for 35 to 45 minutes, stirring after about 20 minutes, then checking after another 15 minutes. (Note that if you use maple syrup rather than date syrup, baking time may increase to 5 or 10 minutes longer.) The granola should be dry and darker, and the nuts should be nicely

(Continued on page 62)

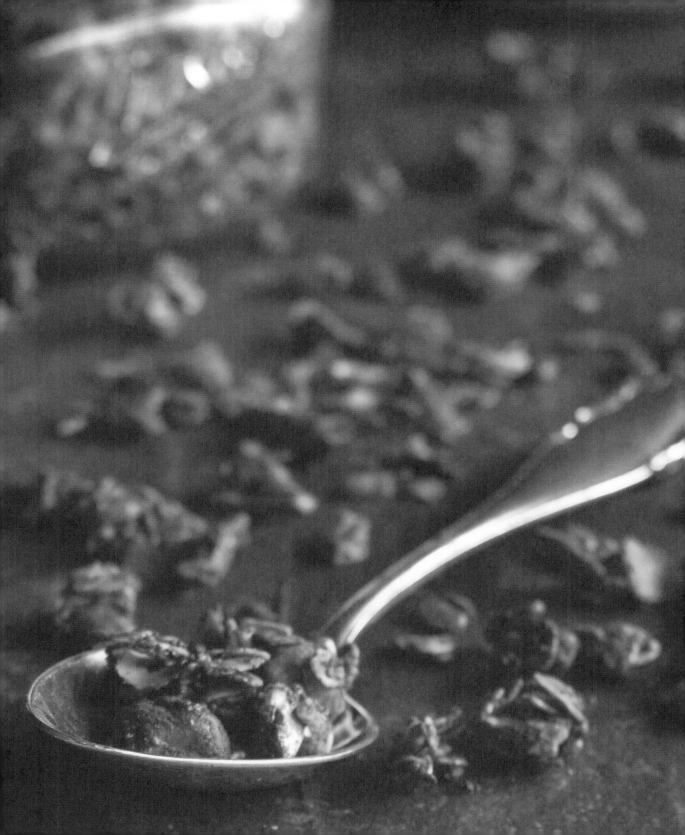

roasted. The granola will crisp up as it cools. Let the granola sit on the pans and cool completely. Once it's cooled, stir in dried fruit or cocoa nibs.

⅔ cup mixed dried fruit (dried cherries, dried blueberries, raisins, dried cranberries, goji berries, chopped dried apricots, chopped dates, etc.) and/or cocoa nibs

Store in airtight containers. It stays fresh for 2 to 3 weeks.

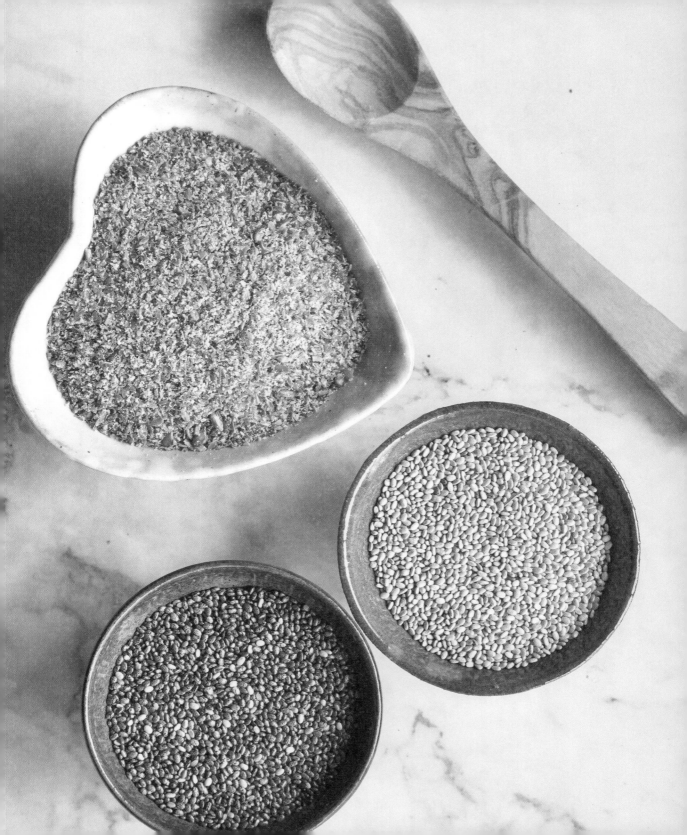

Gingerbread Steel-Cut Oats with Pears

Makes 4 servings

Steel-cut oats are denser and chewier than rolled oats, which make them more filling, because our digestive systems have to work harder and longer to break them down. The molasses, ginger, and cinnamon create a classic gingerbread flavor for this dish. As a special touch, I top my oats with fresh pear cubes, slices, or cooked compote—the combination is out-of-this-world good. If you have Irish or Scottish oats in your cupboard, feel free to substitute them for the steel-cut oats.

Pressure cooker directions. Add the following ingredients to an electric pressure cooker. Lock the lid. Move the knob to "Sealing." Use the "Multigrain," "Manual," "Pressure Cook," or "High" mode and set for 6 minutes. Wait for 10 minutes after the pressure cooker is done, then move the knob to "Venting" and release the remaining steam before opening the lid.

- **3¾ cups water**
- **1 cup steel-cut oats**
- **2 tablespoons flaxseed meal**
- **3 tablespoons date syrup or maple syrup**
- **2 tablespoons mild molasses**
- **2–3 teaspoons finely chopped fresh ginger**
- **1½ teaspoons cinnamon**
- **1 teaspoon vanilla extract or vanilla powder**
- **¼ teaspoon ground cloves**
- **⅛ teaspoon salt (optional)**

After opening the lid, stir the oats. They are ready to eat. Top with one or more of the following toppings.

- **2 ripe pears, diced or sliced**
- **Nondairy milk**
- **Walnuts, almonds, pecans, or other nuts**

The gingerbread oats will keep in the refrigerator for about a week. They also freeze well.

Stovetop directions. The night before or at least 2 hours before serving, in a large saucepan bring 4 cups of water to a boil. Turn off the heat. Add in all ingredients above (except the toppings) and stir. Cover the pan and let it stand for 2 hours or overnight. After 2 hours or in the morning, bring the mixture to a boil, reduce to low, and simmer until the grains are tender, 10 to 15 minutes. Add more water if needed.

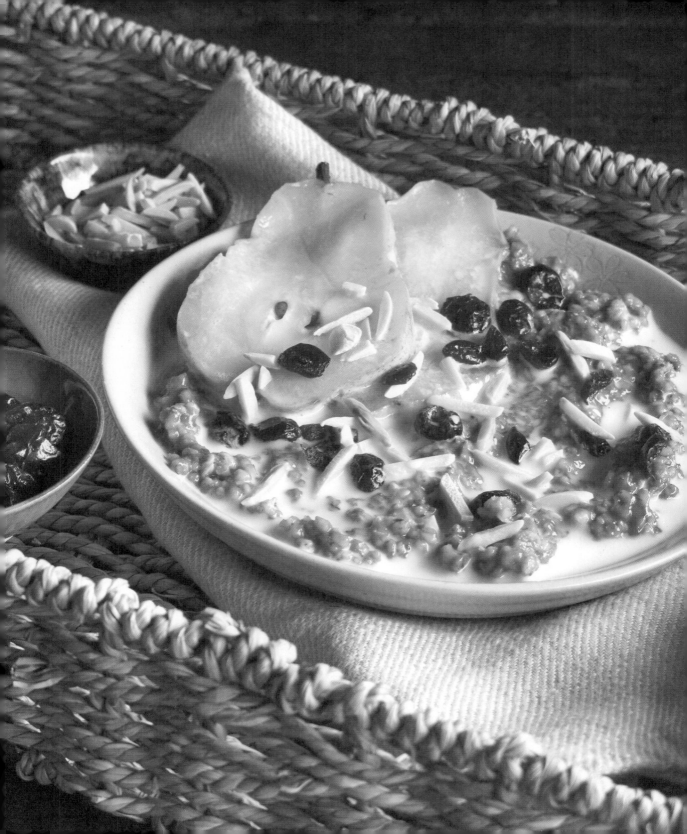

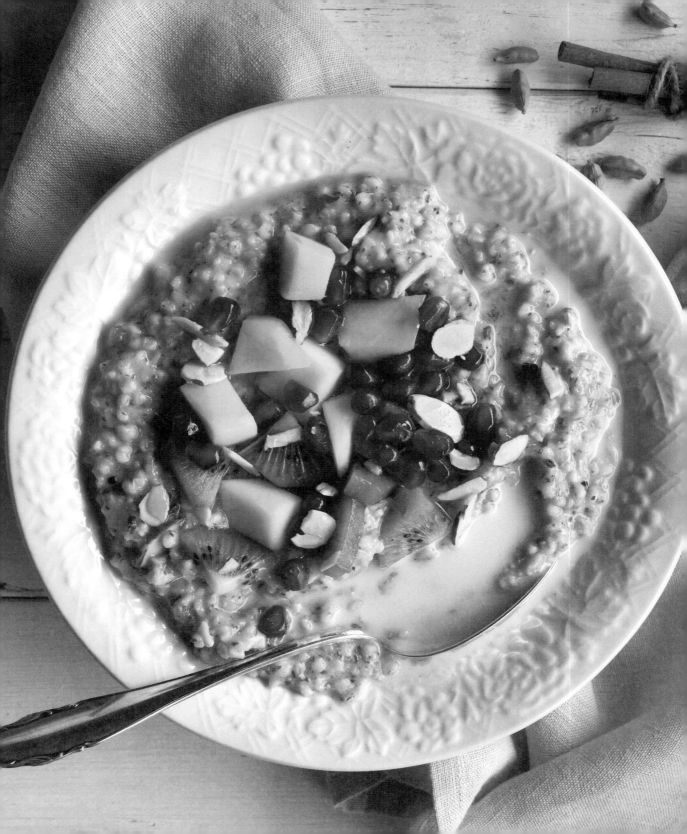

Chai-Spiced Steel-Cut Oats

Makes 4 servings

Warm and comforting on a cold morning, this dish is also packed with protein, complex carbohydrates, fiber, and a whole lot of antioxidants from the spices. If chai spices aren't your thing, you can forgo them and substitute your favorites. I tried using ground spices, but the result wasn't nearly as flavorful. Once you have cinnamon sticks, cardamom seeds, and fresh ginger on hand, this recipe is a snap. If you don't have a pressure cooker, I highly recommend the overnight stovetop method provided. It works so much better than boiling the oats all at once.

Pressure cooker directions. Add the following ingredients to an electric pressure cooker. Lock the lid. Move the knob to "Sealing." Use the "Multigrain," "Pressure Cook," "Manual," or "High" mode and set for 6 minutes. Wait for 10 minutes after the pressure cooker is done, then move the knob to "Venting" and release the remaining steam before opening the lid.

3¾ cups water
1 cup steel-cut oats
¼ cup flaxseed meal
1 tablespoon finely chopped fresh ginger
2 cinnamon sticks
Seeds from 6 cardamom pods or ¾ teaspoon cardamom seeds or ground cardamom
⅛ teaspoon salt (optional)
5–10 grinds fresh black pepper

After opening the lid, stir the oats and remove the cinnamon sticks. The oats are ready to eat. Top with one or more of the following toppings.

Plant-based milk
Fresh or dried fruit
Chopped walnuts or other nuts
Hemp seeds
Sweetener (date sugar, date paste, banana, or other)

The oats will keep in the refrigerator for about a week. They also freeze well.

Stovetop directions. The night before or at least 2 hours before serving, in a large saucepan bring 4 cups of water to a boil. Turn off the heat. Add in all ingredients above (except the toppings) and stir. Cover the pan and let it stand for 2 hours or overnight. After 2 hours or in the morning, bring the mixture to a boil, reduce to low, and simmer until the grains are tender, 10 to 15 minutes. Add more water if needed.

Kale and Berry Detox Smoothie

Makes 1 large smoothie

Yes, there are a gazillion smoothie recipes out there, but I love this one when I want a seriously healthy drink. It's full of antioxidants and other anti-inflammatory compounds. The citrus and ginger give it a zing that will keep you drinking more and more. I was surprised it didn't need any sweetener, but add some if you need it. It also keeps well in the fridge for the next day. Don't be put off by the dark color—the anti-inflammatory anthocyanins are at work!

Add the following ingredients to a blender and blend until smooth. Add more liquid if needed.

- **Juice from 1 orange (or ½ cup orange juice)**
- **Juice from ½ large lemon or 1 small lemon (about 1½ tablespoons)**
- **1½ cups mixed fresh or frozen berries or other fruit of your choice**
- **1 packed cup chopped kale leaves (chopped stems are okay to include)**
- **½ cup water or cold chamomile tea**
- **1½ tablespoons chopped fresh ginger**

This smoothie can be made ahead and frozen. When ready to drink it, defrost it in the microwave for 30 to 60 seconds, and, for best results, blend it again briefly.

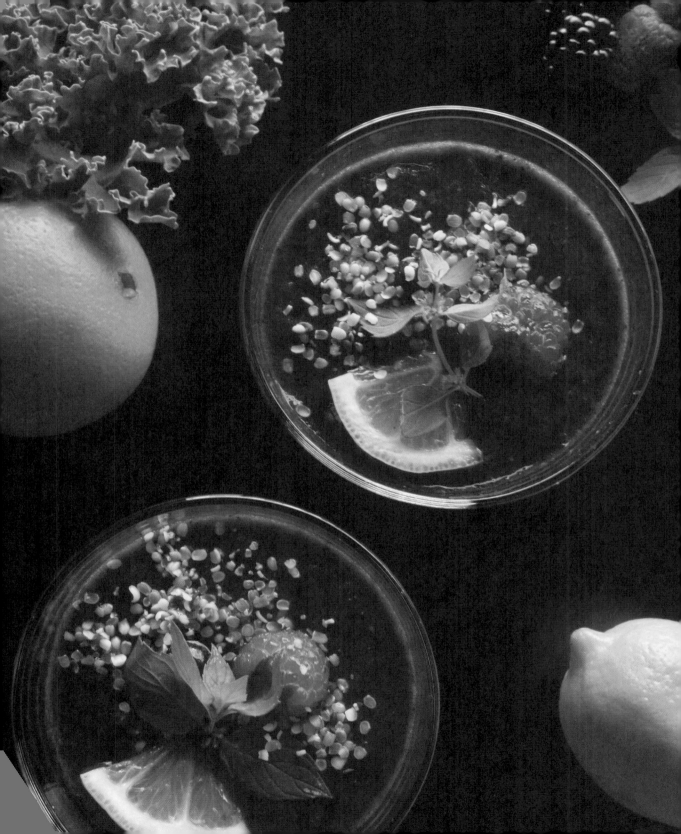

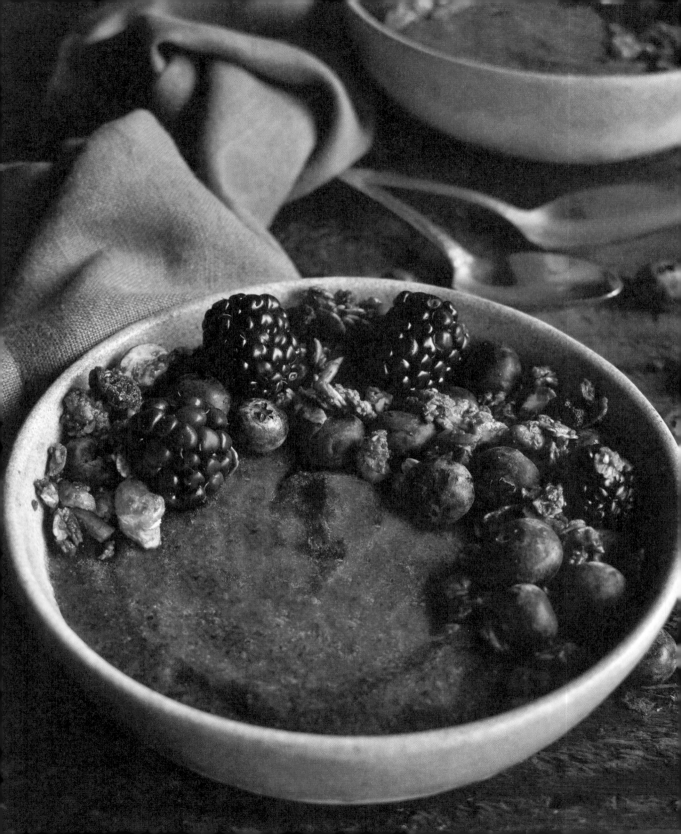

Daily Habit Berry Smoothie Bowl

Makes 4 smoothie bowls

I made up this recipe when I decided to eat half a cup of berries every day. The consensus among nutritional experts about the benefits of berries is too strong to ignore, and berries are anti-inflammatory superstars. If fresh berries aren't available, I make a batch of these smoothie bowls, eat one bowlful that morning, and freeze the remaining servings. For the next three days, I pop one of the frozen bowls in the microwave, then stir with a fork. I love my smoothie bowl with a spoonful of unsweetened soy milk yogurt and a sprinkling of Orange-Spice Granola (page 60).

Blend the following ingredients together in a blender until smooth.

2 cups frozen berries (I prefer blueberries)

1½ cups water or cold chamomile tea or more, if needed

1 banana, sliced and frozen

¼ cup flaxseed meal

¾ teaspoon ginger powder or more, if needed

Sweetener of choice (optional)

These smoothie bowls are ready to eat. You can freeze them in individual portions for eating later.

Matcha Mango Freezer-Prep Smoothie

Makes 1 smoothie

Matcha—a green tea powder and anti-inflammatory superstar—makes for a great smoothie ingredient with its bright color and high nutritional value. I especially love the color combination with mangoes. This smoothie is designed for easy prep. You can freeze most of the ingredients days or weeks ahead of time in a container or bag. When you're ready for a smoothie, just add water and lemon juice, blend, and drink.

Add the following ingredients to a blender and blend until smooth. Add more water if needed.

- **1 banana, sliced and frozen**
- **1 cup frozen mango cubes**
- **½ packed cup fresh spinach leaves**
- **1 tablespoon flaxseed meal**
- **1 teaspoon matcha tea powder**
- **½ teaspoon ginger powder**
- **¼ teaspoon turmeric**
- **1⅓ cups water or cold chamomile tea or more, if needed**
- **½ tablespoon freshly squeezed lemon juice**

This smoothie is ready to drink. To prep multiple smoothies at the same time, freeze the solid ingredients together in a plastic bag or freezer-safe container. To make the smoothie, empty the contents of the frozen bag or container into the blender, add in the liquid ingredients, and blend.

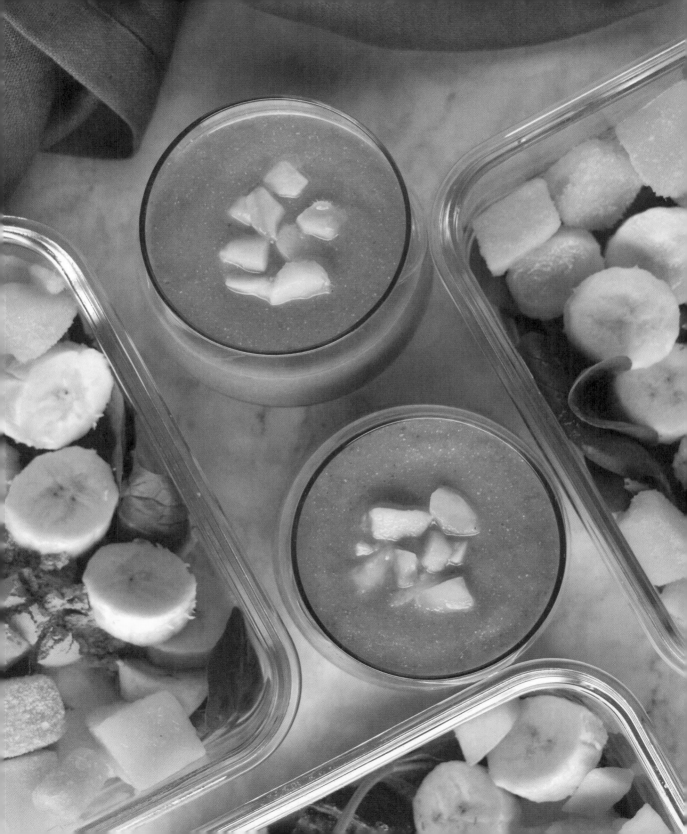

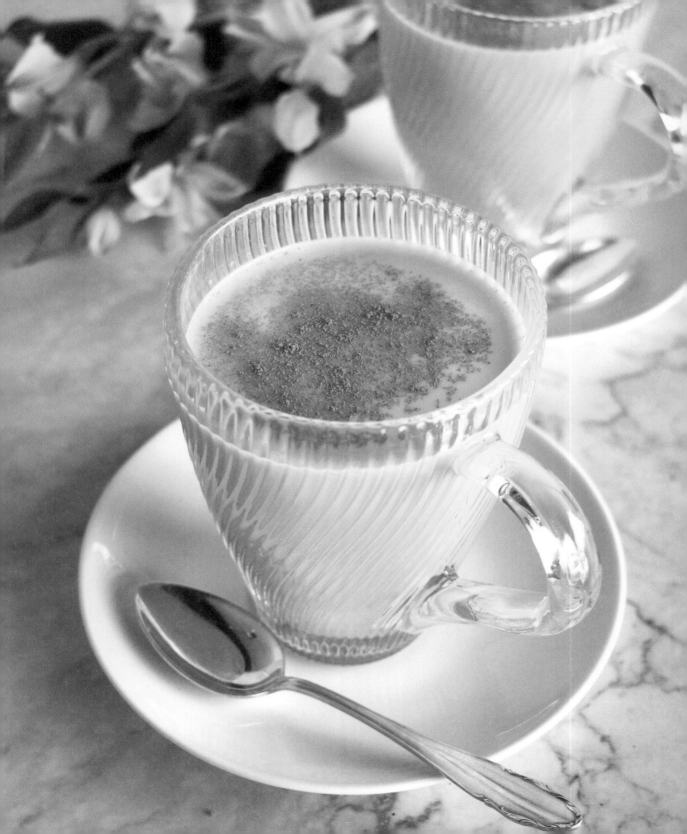

Creamy Turmeric Tea

Makes 2 servings

I can still remember my first cup of turmeric tea at a local Portland tearoom. What a revelation! After I created my own method for making turmeric tea, my sister tested the recipe for me and found a few days later that she was craving more of it. Locating some of the ingredients might take a little effort if you don't already have them, but once you have a stock of them, you'll have enough for many batches. You can use the cinnamon stick up to five times—just rinse it and let it dry on a towel.

Stir together the following ingredients in a medium saucepan and slowly bring the mixture to a boil over low-medium heat. As soon as it boils, turn off the heat and let the mixture steep for at least a minute, up to 5 minutes.

1 cup water
1–2 black tea bags (depending on how strong you want the tea to be)
1"–1½" piece fresh ginger, peeled, grated, and thinly sliced or finely chopped
8 black peppercorns or ⅛ teaspoon roughly ground pepper
2 cardamom pods, crushed with the side of a knife, or ¼ teaspoon seeds
1 cinnamon stick or ⅛ teaspoon ground cinnamon
1 teaspoon turmeric

After the tea has steeped to your liking, add the following ingredients and bring the mixture back up to steaming, not quite boiling.

2 cups nondairy milk*
1 tablespoon maple syrup or other sweetener

This tea is ready to drink. Taste for sweetness and adjust. Pour the tea through a strainer into a teapot or directly into 2 cups. The tea can be made ahead and refrigerated for up to 3 to 4 days, just warm it up when you are ready to drink it. It does not freeze well.

---

* If you have a milk steamer, you can make this a turmeric latte by adding steamed milk to the steeped and sweetened tea.

Chamomile Ginger Tonic Tea

Makes 1 serving

Made with 100 percent anti-inflammatory superstars, this tea is healing and calming. It has no caffeine and could become a favorite after-dinner drink when you want to distract yourself from sweets. It's also perfect for soothing a sore throat. You can adjust the elements to suit your taste, especially more mint or ginger, or substitute orange for lemon. This recipe can be doubled or tripled for tea with friends.

Prep the ginger. To release some of the juices, put the ginger slices on a cutting board and crush them with the side of a chef's knife or with the bottom of a glass. You can also top them with wax paper and tap them gently with a mallet or hammer.

6 dime-size slices peeled fresh ginger

Make the tea. Boil 12 to 16 ounces of water in a small saucepan. Once it boils, turn off the heat and remove the pan from the stove. Add the following ingredients and let them steep for 5 to 8 minutes.

The ginger slices
1 chamomile teabag or 1 heaping teaspoon loose dried chamomile tea
1 small lemon slice with peel
1 sprig fresh mint or spearmint or ½ teaspoon dried mint

Once the tea is brewed to your liking, set a strainer on top of a teacup and pour the tea through the strainer. You may want to keep the lemon slice for your tea.

Options

Skip the saucepan and brew the tea in a small teapot or directly in your cup. Leave the ingredients in the tea as you sip.

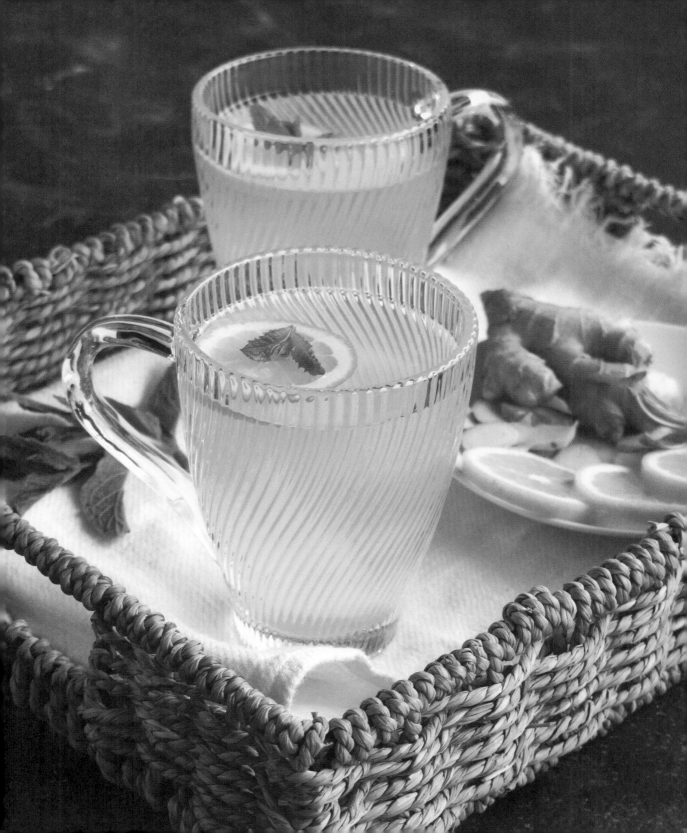

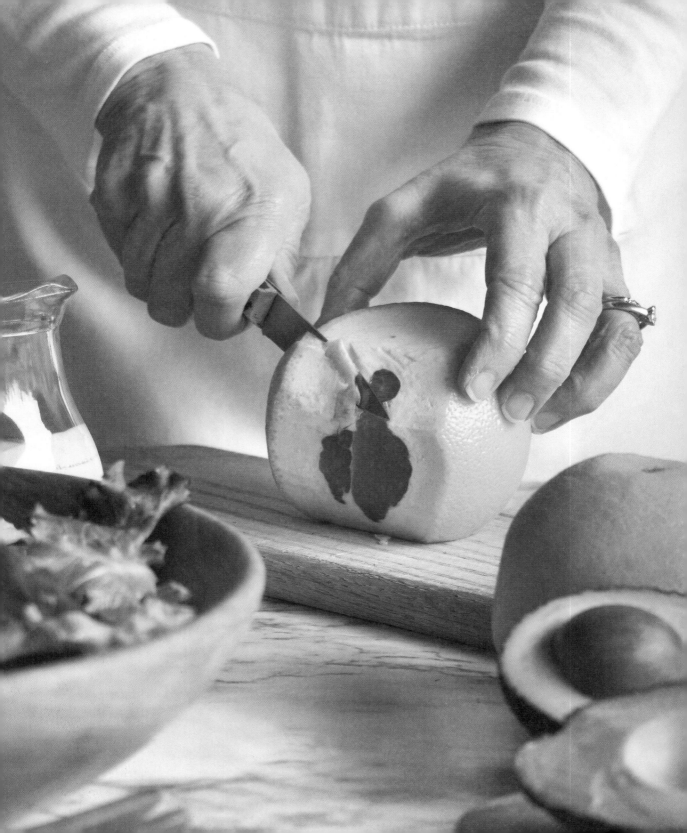

Salads

I grew up with iceberg lettuce salads topped with French dressing made from a packet. I count myself fortunate to have eaten a salad virtually every night as a kid—what a great preparation for appreciating greens for the rest of my life.

As I expanded my gastronomic horizons, I discovered the wide variety of greens and lettuces I could use, and I found out about salads from other cultures. I could add fruit, nuts, grains, and legumes to my salads, too! I particularly love a chopped salad with ingredients that don't wilt after being dressed—these salads can last several days in the fridge and are usually hearty enough to serve as an entree.

So many anti-inflammatory superstars work in salads, including red peppers, celery, apples, pomegranates, citrus, cherries, cruciferous vegetables, and fiber-filled whole grains and legumes. I like to fuel up at least once a day with a substantial salad.

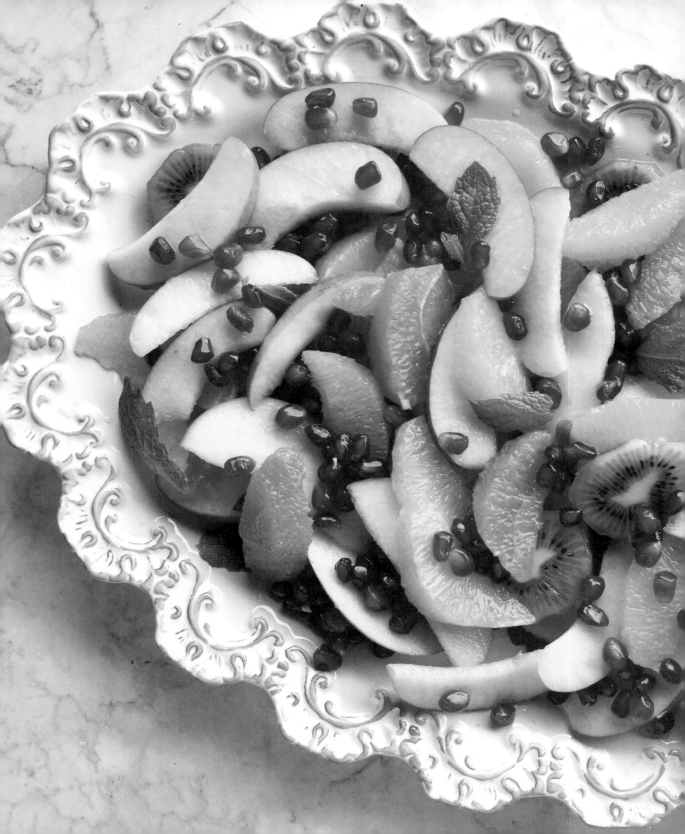

Fruit Salad with a Hint of Ginger

Makes 6 servings

What a difference a small amount of concentrated orange-ginger syrup can make! In general, I don't add anything to fruit salads, but after I tried combining orange and ginger as a syrup for fruit salad, I was convinced that it intensified the fruit flavors. The syrup goes well with any fruit, but since this cookbook is all about calming inflammation, I recommend as many anti-inflammatory superstar ingredients as possible.

Make the ginger syrup. Stir the following ingredients together in a small saucepan. Bring the mixture to a boil, then lower to a simmer and cook, uncovered, until the syrup is medium thick, 15 to 20 minutes. You'll have about ⅓ cup syrup.

> **Juice from 2 oranges (¾ cup)**
> **1½ tablespoons maple syrup**
> **1 tablespoon fresh ginger, thinly sliced**

Let the syrup cool completely. Remove the ginger with a slotted spoon and discard (or use it with a bag of chamomile to make a delicious cup of tea).

Make the salad. Cut up your favorite fruits for a total of 6 cups of fruit.

Apples	**Oranges**
Bananas	**Papayas**
Berries	**Peaches**
Cherries	**Pears**
Grapes (purple or black)	**Plums**
Kiwis	**Pomegranate seeds**
Mangos	**Star fruit**
Melons	

When you are ready to serve this salad, gently toss the orange-ginger syrup with the fruit. The salad will last in the refrigerator for 1 to 2 days. It does not freeze well.

Cherry Waldorf Salad

Makes 5 servings

My mom made Waldorf salad for us quite often. When I was growing up in California, I had no idea a Waldorf Astoria Hotel existed—the name "Waldorf" just sounded kind of exotic to me. In this salad, the sweetness of apples and raisins stands out brilliantly against the faint saltiness and acidity of celery and mayonnaise. The addition of fresh cherries in the summer makes this salad very special and even more anti-inflammatory than it already is.

Stir together the following ingredients in a medium mixing bowl or salad bowl.

2 medium apples (red and unpeeled for anti-inflammatory effect), cored and diced

3 celery stalks, chopped or sliced

⅓ cup dried cranberries or raisins

⅓ cup walnuts, chopped

⅓ cup vegan mayonnaise (try an oil-free plant-based recipe for mayonnaise on graciousvegan.com)

Gently stir in the cherries right before serving (otherwise their color will bleed onto the apples).

1 cup fresh cherries, pitted and halved or quartered

Taste and add sweetener if you need it.

1 or more teaspoons maple syrup (optional)

This salad is ready to eat but can be made 1 to 2 hours in advance and then served. It will keep for 2 to 3 days in the refrigerator. It does not freeze well.

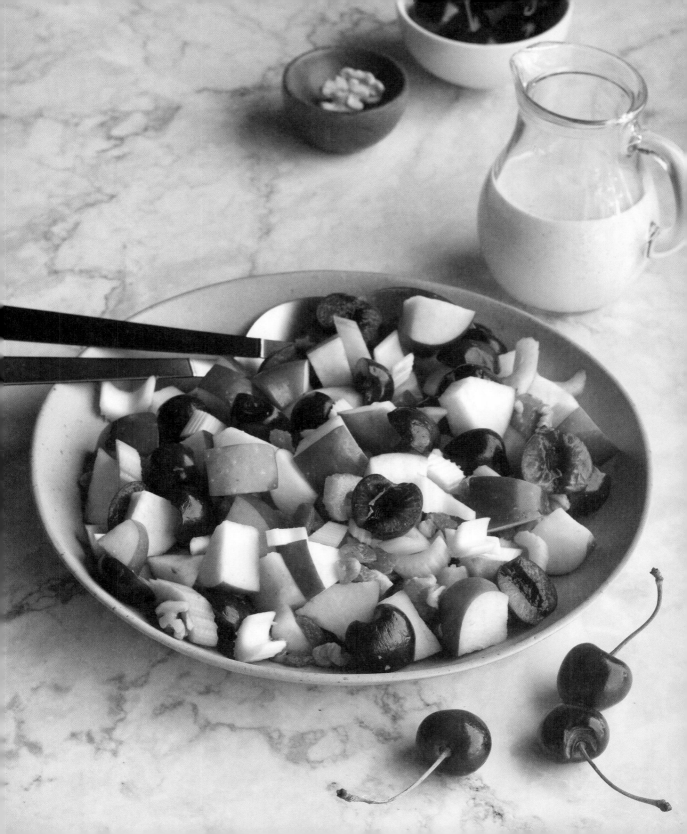

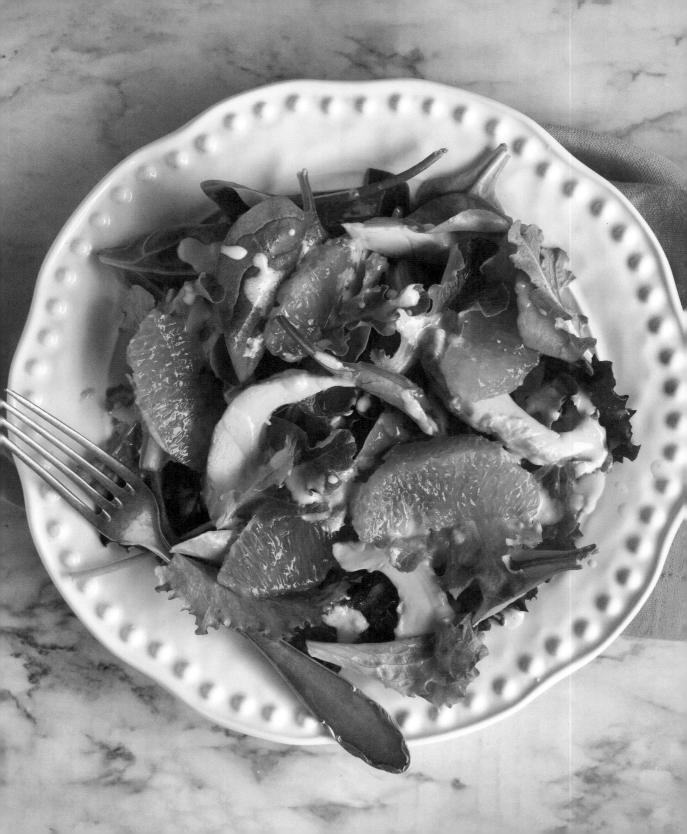

Grapefruit and Avocado Salad

Makes 4 servings

The dressing for this salad was a particular hit with my recipe testers. They decided they wanted to use it on lots of different salads, not just this one. When grapefruits are in season, combining them with avocado and greens makes for a spectacular salad—both in color and taste. The technique I use to prepare the grapefruits is called "supreming" (cutting away the skin and then the membranes), resulting in perfect segments without the chewiness.

Prep the grapefruit. First, use a zester to generate grapefruit zest. Set aside.

1 teaspoon zest from 1 large ruby red or pink grapefruit

Then, slice off the top and bottom of the whole grapefruit so that the grapefruit sits still on a cutting board. Hold the grapefruit steady and cut away the skin and white pith on all sides, then slice in between the segments and membranes to free the segments. Squeeze grapefruit juice from the membrane remainders.

2 tablespoons grapefruit juice

Make the dressing. Whisk the following ingredients together in a bowl or blend them in a small blender.

The 1 teaspoon grapefruit zest
The 2 tablespoons grapefruit juice
2 tablespoons tahini
2 tablespoons water
2 teaspoons white wine vinegar, champagne vinegar, or sherry vinegar (see box on page 88)
1 teaspoon Dijon mustard
¼ teaspoon salt (or to taste)

Assemble the salad. Put the following ingredients in a salad bowl.

4–5 cups spring mix, spinach, or cut or torn leaf lettuce
The grapefruit segments
1 avocado, peeled and sliced or cubed
A handful of roasted nuts or seeds (optional)

Add about half the dressing to the salad bowl and gently toss everything together. Add more dressing if needed. The salad is ready to serve and will keep for about an hour. It does not freeze well.

Spinach and Apple Salad with Curry Dressing

🌿

Makes 4 servings

Apple and spinach go very well with curry flavors, as do raisins and peanuts. You can substitute your favorite fruits, greens, dried fruit, and nuts, but this particular combination is worth trying at least once. For an entree salad, add cooked grains and/or beans. This salad pairs well with Curried Amaranth Patties (page 161) or Vegetable Tikka Masala Curry (page 213).

Make the dressing. Blend the following ingredients together in a small blender.

3 tablespoons almond butter

3 tablespoons water

2 tablespoons silken tofu or 1 tablespoon tahini mixed with 1 tablespoon water

2 tablespoons sherry vinegar, champagne vinegar, or white wine vinegar (see box on page 88)

1½ teaspoons maple syrup

½ teaspoon curry powder

¼ teaspoon ginger powder

¼ teaspoon turmeric

¼ teaspoon salt (or to taste)

⅛ teaspoon freshly ground black pepper (or to taste)

Make the salad. Toss together the following ingredients in a salad bowl.

5 ounces baby spinach

1 red apple, unpeeled, diced or sliced

⅓ cup roasted peanuts

¼ cup golden or black raisins

4 green onions, sliced

Add about half the dressing to the salad, toss together, and add more dressing as needed, or serve the salad on individual plates and let each person add their own dressing. The salad is ready to serve. It will last 1 to 2 days in the refrigerator. It does not freeze well.

(Continued on page 88)

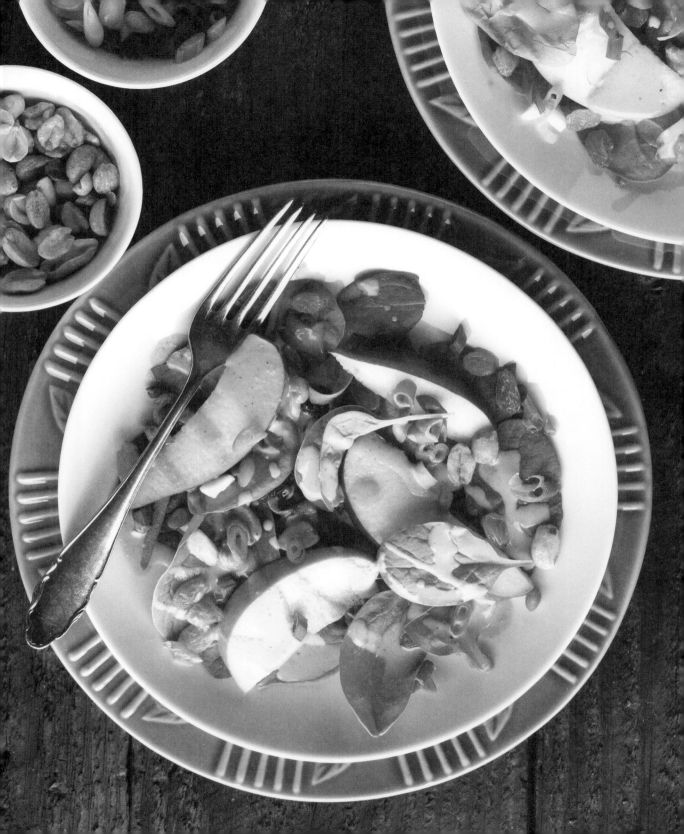

Celebrating vinegar!

There are many types of vinegar, and since most of us have limited cupboard space, we need to decide on just a few. Apple cider vinegar and distilled white vinegar are staples, and most people also keep balsamic vinegar. The vinegars I call for in this recipe and a few others are lighter and milder in flavor than the three most common vinegars. Champagne vinegar offers a mellow, delicate flavor, while sherry vinegar is slightly nutty. White and red wine vinegars are milder than distilled white vinegar and less fruity than apple cider vinegar. All of them don't steal the show like balsamic vinegar can, with its complex, sweet taste. If you make a lot of homemade dressings, I recommend having at least one of these lighter, milder vinegars on hand.

Apple and Greens
with Candied Walnuts

Makes 5 servings

Making a vinaigrette without oil is tricky. I find that almond butter is the best substitute for this dressing. After blending the almond butter with vinegar, water, and other ingredients, it smooths out like oil in a thick emulsion. The candied walnuts add a special touch to this salad, although you could leave them out for a simpler and quicker dish. This salad pairs well with many entrees, including Stuffed Bell Pepper Rings (page 199) and Baked Penne with Bell Peppers and Ricotta (page 222).

Make the candied walnuts. Preheat the oven to 350°F. Line a sheet pan with parchment paper or a silicone mat. Toast the walnuts on the pan until fragrant and just golden, 5 to 7 minutes.

⅔ cup raw walnut halves or pieces

Meanwhile, combine the following ingredients in a small bowl and set aside.

½ teaspoon curry powder
⅛ teaspoon cumin
⅛ teaspoon salt (or to taste)

Once the walnuts are toasted, bring the following ingredients to a boil in a small skillet.

1 tablespoon maple syrup
2 teaspoons water

Add in the toasted walnuts, stirring to coat. Simmer until no liquid remains, about 3 minutes, then add in the dry spice mixture and toss to coat well. Spread the coated nuts on the same baking sheet used earlier to toast the nuts and roast them until the coating is dry and slightly golden, about 5 minutes. Let the nuts cool on the pan.

Make the dressing. Whisk the following ingredients together in a bowl or blend them in a small blender.

¼ cup almond butter
¼ cup water
¼ cup balsamic vinegar
2 teaspoons maple syrup
2 teaspoons Dijon mustard

(Continued on page 91)

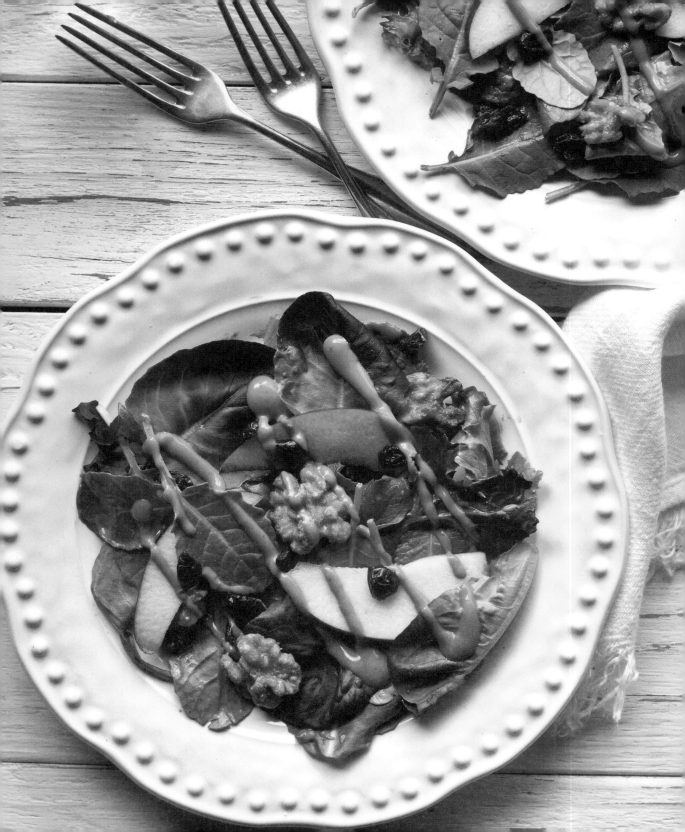

½ teaspoon salt (or to taste)

¼ teaspoon garlic powder

¼ teaspoon basil

¼ teaspoon oregano

Freshly ground black pepper to taste

Finish the salad. Toss together the following ingredients with the dressing in a large bowl or salad bowl. Alternatively, build individual servings on separate salad plates and drizzle the dressing over each.

The candied walnuts

5 ounces spring mix, baby spinach, or other greens

2 red apples, unpeeled, thinly sliced

⅓ cup dried cherries or cranberries

Once dressed, the salad will last an hour or 2. Undressed, the salad will last 1 to 2 days. It does not freeze well.

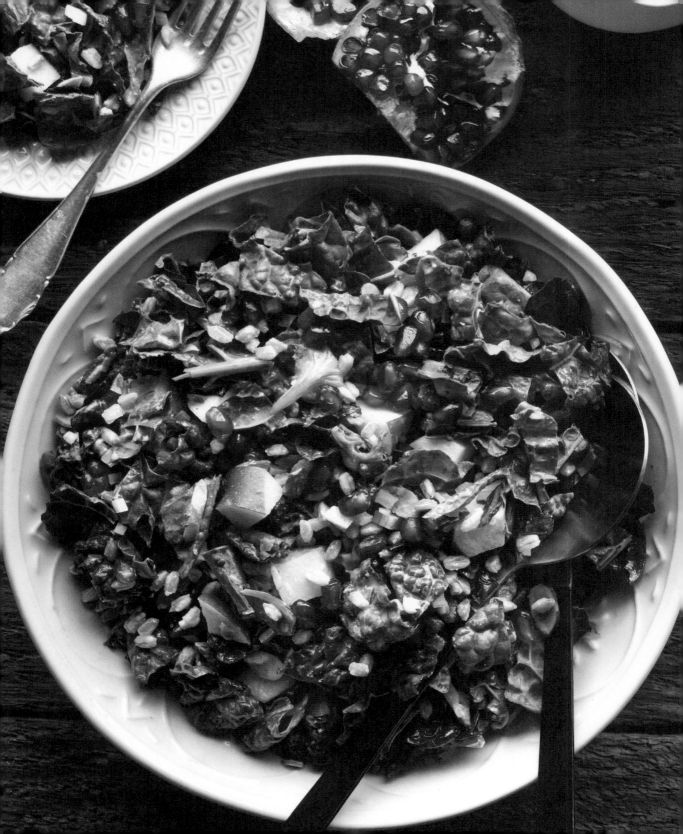

Chopped Salad
with Orange Vinaigrette

Makes 8 servings

This salad makes a great addition to a winter holiday dinner—the green kale and red fruits are perfect for the season. In spring, you could substitute spinach, blanched asparagus, radishes, and snow peas or sugar snap peas. My favorite grain for chopped salads is farro, but many other grains work well in this salad. Since the kale doesn't wilt in a salad like this, you can plan on eating leftovers for a couple of days afterward.

Make the vinaigrette. Blend the following ingredients together in a small blender or whisk them together in a bowl.

> 3 tablespoons champagne vinegar, sherry vinegar, or white wine vinegar (see box on page 88)
> 2 tablespoons tahini
> 2 tablespoons fresh orange juice
> 1½ tablespoons maple syrup or date syrup
> ½ teaspoon orange zest
> ⅛ teaspoon salt (or to taste)
> Freshly ground black pepper to taste

Make the salad. Add the following ingredients to a large bowl and toss with half of the dressing. This part of the salad can sit and absorb the dressing for at least 10 minutes whereas the final ingredients should be kept aside until the end.

> 1 small bunch (6 cups) kale, destemmed and chopped into small pieces
> 1 cup cooked farro, brown rice, quinoa, spelt, or other whole grain
> ¼ cup shallot or red onion, diced or thinly sliced

Add the final ingredients right before serving and add as much of the remaining dressing as you like.

> 1 small red apple, unpeeled and diced and/or ½ cup pomegranate seeds
> 3 tablespoons dried cherries or cranberries
> 3 tablespoons roasted nuts (I prefer pecans, almonds, or walnuts)
> Additional dressing as needed

This salad will last several days in the refrigerator. It does not freeze well.

Italian Chopped Salad
with Sun-Dried Tomato Dressing

Makes 4 large servings or 8 small servings

Sun-dried tomatoes aren't as popular as they once were, but they still deserve to shine. Their strong flavor dominates this dressing, but the salad offers other high-volume flavor options like radicchio, red onions, and Kalamata olives that stand up well against the sun-dried tomatoes. I love cooked grains in chopped salads to make them hearty enough to be the centerpiece of lunch or dinner, so feel free to add grains if you like.

Make the dressing. Blend the following ingredients together in a blender.

1¼ cups water
½ cup dried sun-dried tomatoes, each cut into a few pieces*
¼ cup tahini
¼ cup tofu of choice or cooked white beans
3 tablespoons freshly squeezed lemon juice
1 clove garlic, cut into a few pieces
2 teaspoons nutritional yeast
1 teaspoon basil
½ teaspoon salt (or to taste)
Freshly ground black pepper to taste

Make the salad. Create a mix equaling 8 cups of the following ingredients. Add them to a large mixing bowl or salad bowl.

Romaine lettuce, chopped
Radicchio, chopped
Baby spinach, chopped
Raw or roasted red bell pepper, diced or sliced
Garbanzo beans, drained and rinsed
Red onions, chopped or sliced
Cherry tomatoes, whole or halved

(Continued on page 96)

---

* If your sun-dried tomatoes are old and dry, soak them in warm water for about 20 minutes, then drain them.

The Plant-Based Anti-Inflammatory Cookbook

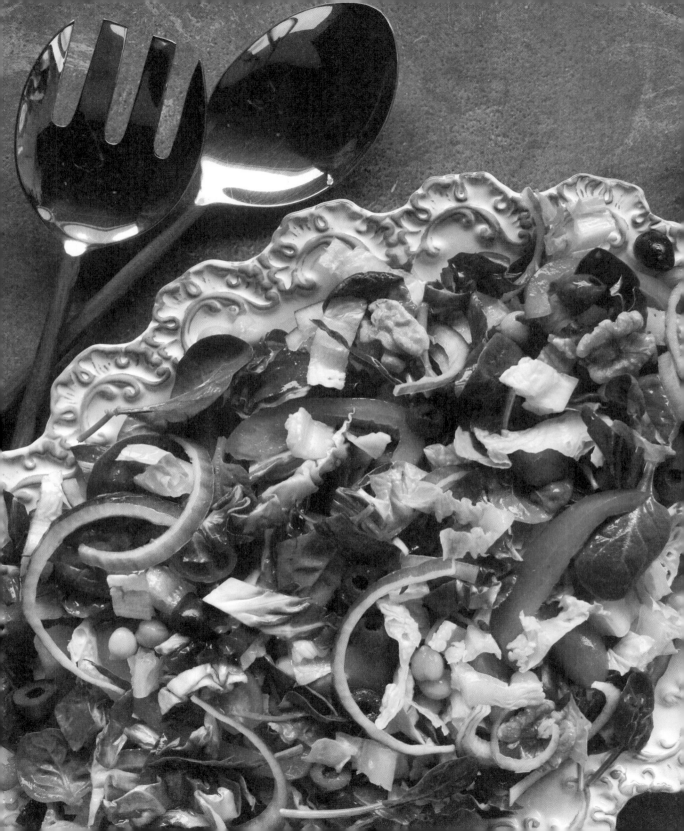

Add the following ingredients to the same bowl and toss everything together.

> **1⅓ cups Greek or Kalamata olives, halved or sliced**
> **½ cup raw or roasted walnuts, roughly chopped**
> **1 cup sun-dried tomato dressing (or more to taste)**

Once dressed, the salad will last an hour or 2. Undressed, the salad will last 3 to 4 days in the refrigerator. It does not freeze well. Leftover dressing will thicken up, so you may need to stir in more water before serving.

Technicolor Tabbouleh Salad

Makes 5 servings

I admit I'm not the biggest fan of tabbouleh salads when the only thing you can taste is parsley. I prefer when the bulgur gets a bit more prominence. There's still plenty of parsley in this rendition, but I bring other colorful ingredients into play to take full advantage of anti-inflammatory superstars. This salad lasts several days in the refrigerator (yay for leftovers!) and goes well with bean soups like Moroccan Chickpea Soup (page 115).

Reconstitute the bulgur. Combine the following ingredients in a bowl. Cover the bowl until the bulgur is tender (20 to 30 minutes). If there is water remaining after the bulgur is tender, pour it off. Fluff the bulgur with a fork.

¾ cup boiling water
½ cup uncooked bulgur wheat

Make the dressing. While the bulgur soaks, whisk the following ingredients together in a bowl or blend them in a small blender.

2 cloves garlic, finely chopped
Juice from 2 lemons (4–6 tablespoons)
2 tablespoons water
2 tablespoons tahini
½ teaspoon cumin
½ teaspoon salt (or to taste)
Freshly ground black pepper to taste

Assemble the salad. Toss the following ingredients together in a large bowl.

The bulgur
The dressing
2 packed cups fresh parsley leaves, minced in the food processor
2 medium tomatoes, diced, or 1½ cups cherry tomatoes, halved or diced
1 large bunch green onions, sliced, or ½ cup red onion, diced
¼ packed cup mint leaves, gently sliced rather than roughly chopped
1 cup cucumber, diced
1 large carrot, grated
1 cup red cabbage, thinly sliced
1 cup red bell pepper, diced

(Continued on page 99)

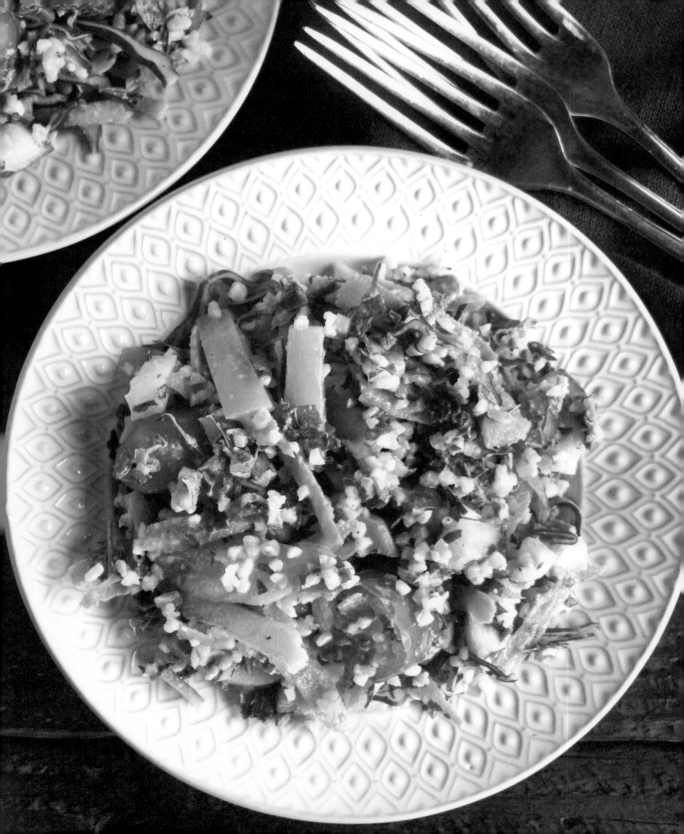

This salad is ready to serve, although it's best after 1 to 2 hours in the refrigerator, when the flavors can blend and the lemon flavor mellows out. Serve at room temperature or chilled. The salad will last several days in the refrigerator. It does not freeze well.

Colorful Coleslaw with Raisins

Makes 4 servings

Coleslaw is a fantastic way to eat one or more servings of a cruciferous vegetable (cabbage)—this recipe's lightly tart dressing brings out cabbage's sweet side. I call for reds, yellows, and greens to complement cabbage's purple hues for a festive, anti-inflammatory take on this humble salad. This dish is perfect for picnics and potlucks. Since the vegan mayonnaise doesn't contain eggs, it has much less risk of spoiling.

Make the dressing. Whisk together the following ingredients in a small bowl.

- ⅓ cup vegan mayonnaise (try an oil-free plant-based recipe for mayonnaise on graciousvegan.com)
- ⅓ cup unsweetened vegan yogurt, sour cream, or cashew cream
- 1 tablespoon maple syrup
- 1 teaspoon apple cider vinegar
- ⅛ teaspoon salt (optional)

Assemble the salad. Toss the following ingredients together in a medium salad bowl.

- The dressing
- 1½ packed cups shredded green cabbage, thinly sliced by hand or in a food processor
- 1½ packed cups shredded red cabbage, thinly sliced by hand or in a food processor
- ½ red bell pepper or 3 mini red peppers, diced
- ½ yellow bell pepper or 3 mini yellow peppers, diced
- 1 medium carrot, grated
- ½ cup dried cherries, dried cranberries, black raisins, or golden raisins

This salad is ready to serve. It will last 1 to 2 days in the refrigerator. It does not freeze well.

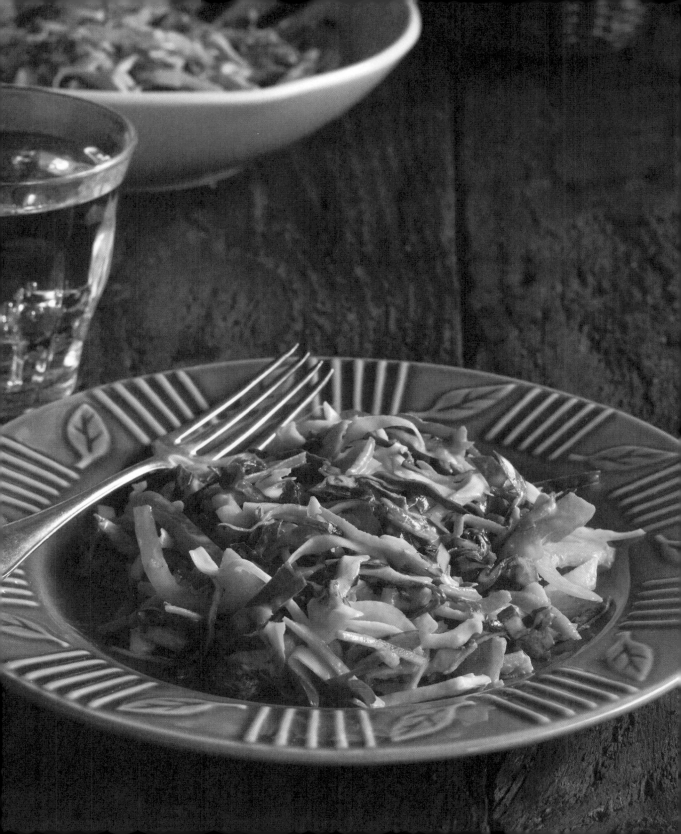

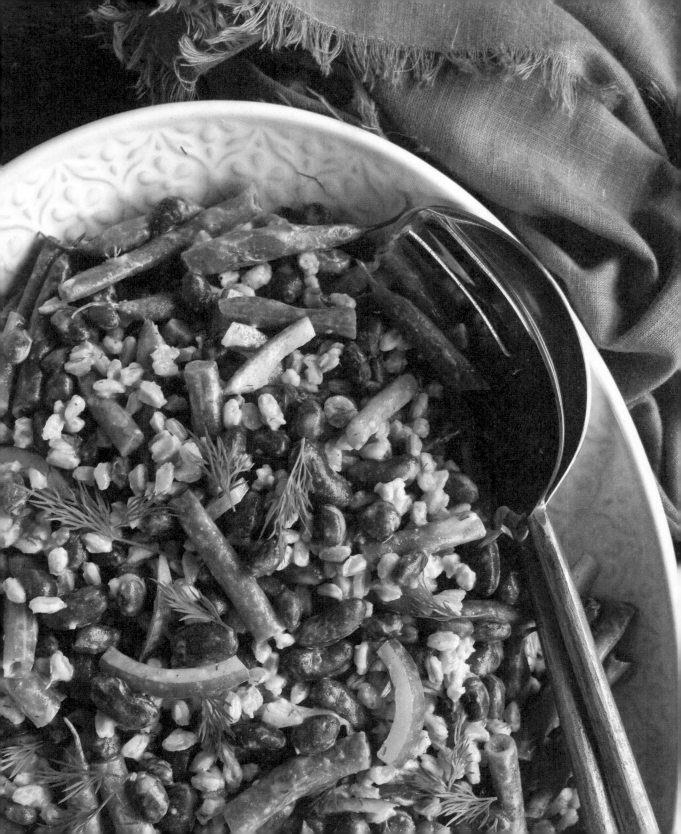

Lemony Farro and Bean Salad

Makes 4 large or 8 small servings

My mom used to whip up a three-bean salad by opening cans of green beans, kidney beans, and garbanzos, then splashing them with oil and vinegar. In this recipe, I still empty a couple cans of beans as she did, but I add grains and omit the oil. Dill and lemon give this salad its signature flavor. I often eat this salad for lunch several days in a row, but it also pairs well with Tomato and Roasted Red Pepper Soup (page 132) for dinner.

Make the dressing. Whisk together the following ingredients in a bowl, jar, or measuring cup.

⅓ cup freshly squeezed lemon juice

2 tablespoons tahini

2 tablespoons water

2 tablespoons fresh dill, chopped, or 2 teaspoons dried dill

2 teaspoons Dijon mustard

¾ teaspoon salt (or to taste)

¼ teaspoon freshly ground black pepper

Make the salad. Add the following ingredients to a large bowl and toss them together until well incorporated.

3 cups trimmed and cut green beans, steamed or boiled to your desired level of tenderness, then immediately drained and dunked into cold water for a few minutes, then drained again

2 cups cooked farro (see the Whole Grains Cooking Guide on page 43; this will require about ¾ cup uncooked farro)

⅓ cup red onion, diced or thinly sliced

1 (15-ounce) can kidney beans or small red beans, drained and rinsed

1 (15-ounce) can black beans, drained and rinsed

Toss about ⅔ of the dressing with the salad. Taste and adjust seasonings and add more dressing as needed. This salad is ready to serve, or you can let it marinate for 1 or 2 hours for a deeper flavor (and less lemon dominance). Serve cold or at room temperature. The salad will last in the refrigerator for 4 to 5 days. It does not freeze well.

Eggless Egg Salad

Makes about 3 cups

This tofu-based egg salad hits the spot in a sandwich, wrap, on celery stalks, or endive leaves. I love it on German-style "Vollkornbrot," that dark, square-shaped bread bursting with whole grains. You can customize the add-ins if you don't like celery, onion, or pickle relish. Paired with a thick soup like Thai-Inspired Creamy Sweet Potato and Lentil Soup (page 119), this salad will create a filling and satisfying meal.

Drain and dry the tofu by wrapping it in paper towels or a clean rag or towel. Lean on the block and firmly squeeze a few times to get out as much water as you can.

1 pound medium-firm or firm tofu

Place the tofu in a medium bowl and mash it into pea-sized chunks with a fork, pastry blender, or potato masher, then stir the following ingredients into the mashed tofu.

⅓ cup vegan mayonnaise (try an oil-free plant-based recipe for mayonnaise on graciousvegan.com)

1 large or 2 small celery stalk(s) and leaves, finely chopped

2 tablespoons red onion, finely chopped

2 tablespoons pickle relish

1 teaspoon turmeric

½ teaspoon kala namak (for more information on kala namak, see box on page 52)

¼ teaspoon salt (or to taste)

Freshly ground pepper to taste

Taste and adjust ingredients as needed. This egg salad is ready to serve. It lasts about a week in the refrigerator. It does not freeze well.

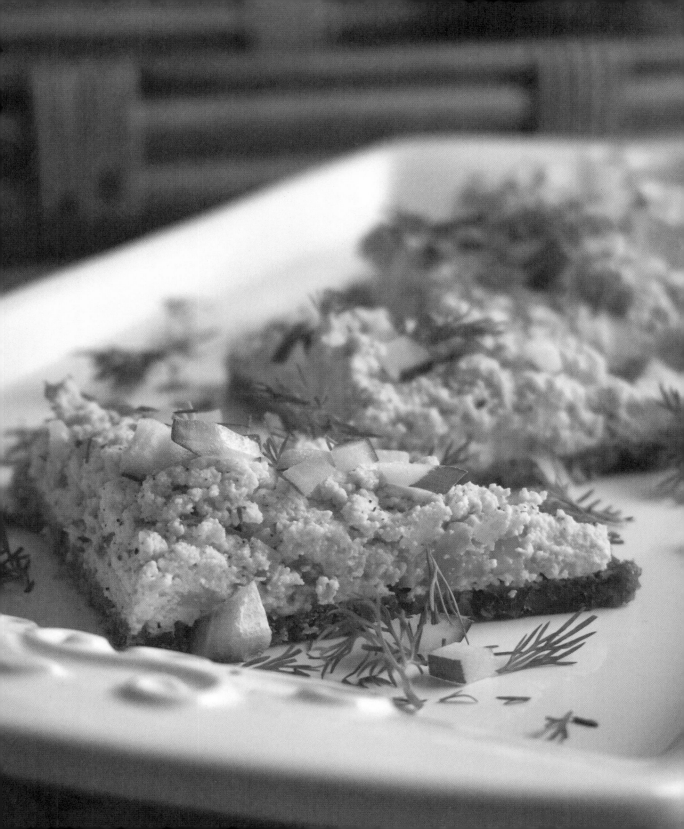

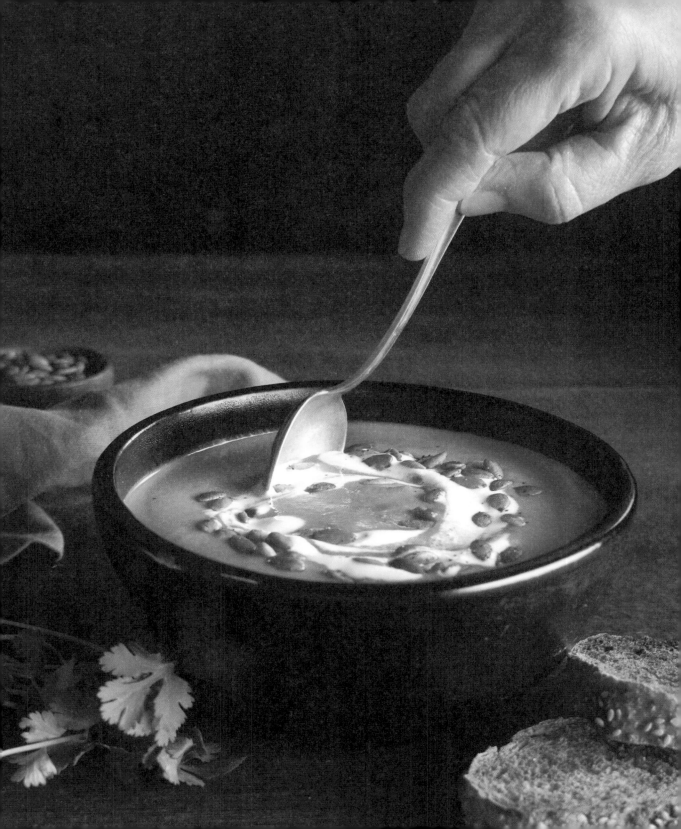

Soups and Stews

The ratio of benefit to effort is almost always high with soups and stews. They taste great, fill you up, yield leftovers, often deliver large doses of nutrients in a concentrated form, and only have two stages, or even just one—add the ingredients to a pot or pressure cooker and let them cook.

I'm particularly fond of bean soups, because getting daily legumes, with their high amounts of fiber, is great for fighting inflammation. I've been known to have Black Bean and Rice Soup (page 121) for lunch and dinner a few days in a row!

Most soups freeze well, meaning these could be a bonus meal in your freezer needing only a salad and fruit or bread to avoid the takeout trap.

When soup's on, healthy, wholesome, anti-inflammatory eating is just around the corner.

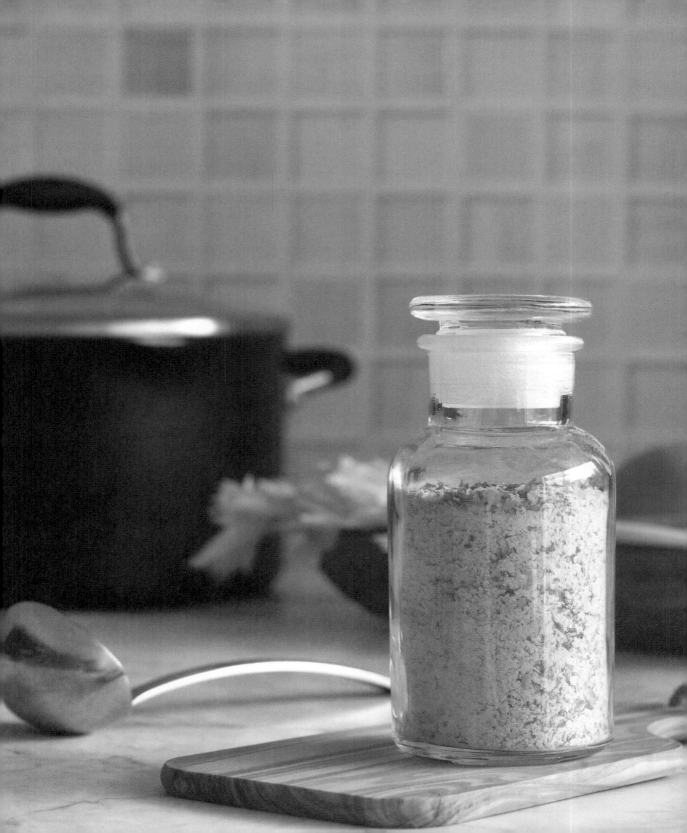

Vegetable Broth Powder

Makes just over 1 cup

I bought vegetable broth powder for years because of the convenience and taste. But the price kept going up and up. So I decided to make my own and I've never looked back. I love this broth for soups, of course, but also for things like rehydrating soy curls. It's also very inexpensive, especially if you get most of your spices and nutritional yeast in the bulk section of a grocery store.

Add the following ingredients to a jar and shake.

- **1 cup nutritional yeast**
- **2 tablespoons garlic powder**
- **2 tablespoons onion powder**
- **4 teaspoons Italian seasoning**
- **1 tablespoon dried parsley flakes**
- **2 teaspoons dried sage**
- **¼ teaspoon turmeric**
- **¼ teaspoon celery seed**
- **¼ teaspoon salt (or to taste)**
- **⅛ teaspoon black pepper**

Use 1 teaspoon vegetable broth powder and 1 cup water for 1 cup vegetable broth. This powder will keep for several months in an airtight container at room temperature.

Creamy Broccoli Soup

Makes 5 servings

This broccoli soup uses nutritional yeast to get that cheesy flavor and cashews for creaminess. It's much healthier than pro-inflammatory restaurant versions made with cream (and sometimes cream cheese). You can use frozen instead of fresh broccoli for a spur-of-the-moment creamy soup. This soup pairs well with Eggless Egg Salad (page 104) on dark bread or Black Bean Burgers (page 197) with all the fixings.

Soak the cashews. Soak the cashews in water for 2 hours or pour boiling water over them, cover, let them soak for about 20 minutes, then drain them. Set aside.

¾ cup raw cashews

Start the soup. Water sauté the onion and garlic in a soup pot or Dutch oven until the onion is tender and transparent, 8 to 10 minutes.

1 small red, yellow, or white onion, diced (about 1 cup)
3 cloves garlic, finely chopped

Add in the following ingredients and stir. Cover the pot and bring to a boil. Once boiling, lower heat to a simmer. Cook about 10 minutes, covered, until the carrots are tender.

1 large carrot, peeled and chopped (about ½ cup)
4 cups broccoli stems and florets, chopped
3 cups vegetable broth
½ teaspoon turmeric
½ teaspoon salt (or to taste)

Finish the cashew cream and the soup. Place the following ingredients in a blender. Blend them on high for 30 seconds or longer, until the cashews are dissolved.

The soaked and drained cashews
2 cups vegetable broth
3 tablespoons yellow or white miso
2 tablespoons nutritional yeast

If your blender is large enough, add the cooked mixture into the blender with the cashew mixture and puree the soup until only small chunks of broccoli and carrot are visible. Alternatively, add the cashew mixture to the pot and use a stick (immersion) blender to puree the soup. Cook the soup on low heat, partially covered, for about 5 minutes until thickened, stirring occasionally so that it doesn't burn on the bottom.

This soup is ready to serve. It will keep well for about a week in the refrigerator. It can be frozen, although the texture and color will not be quite as fresh once thawed.

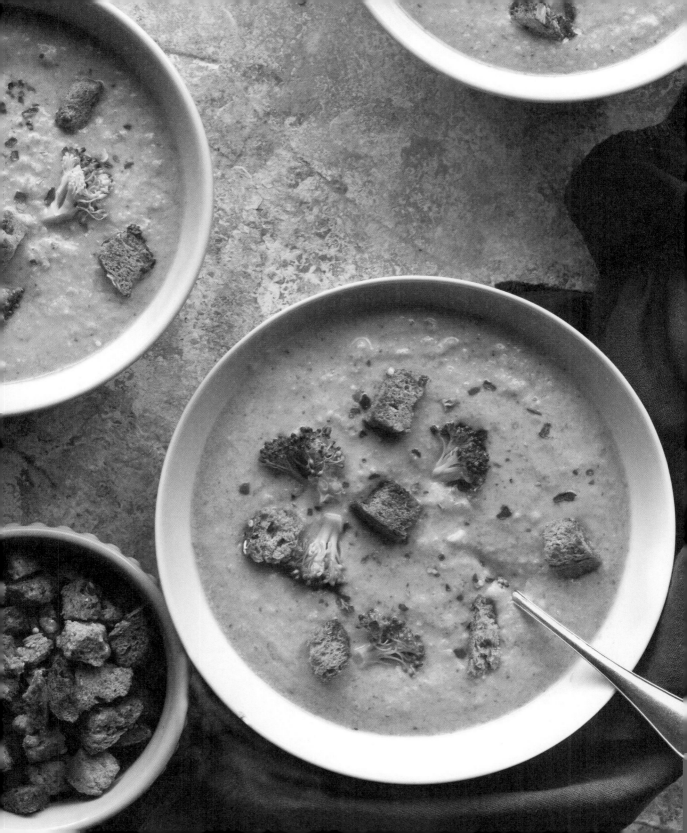

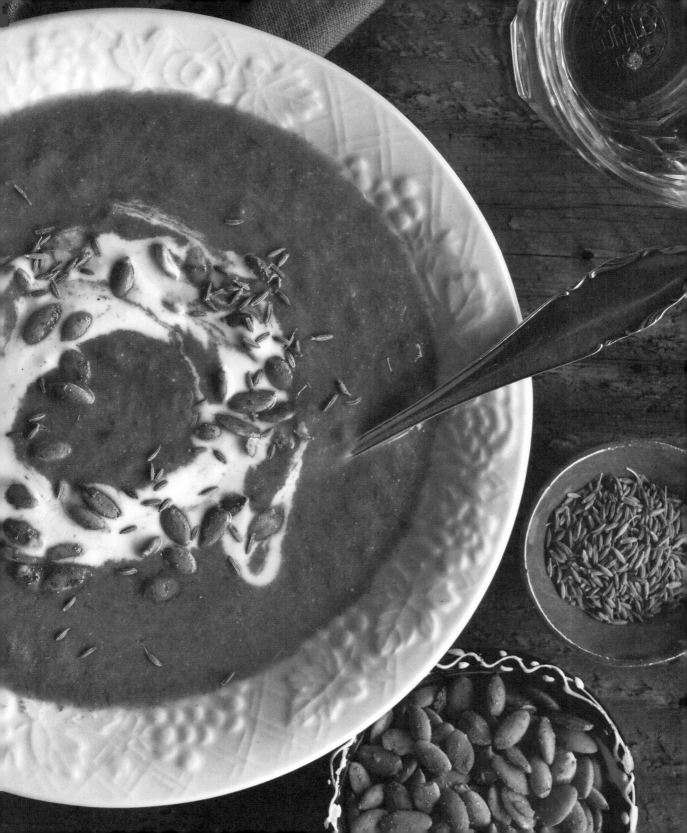

Cream of Spinach Soup

Makes 4 servings

The green color of this soup is mesmerizing. It shouts "Fresh!" A whole pound of spinach is used here, but it quickly shrinks after it hits the hot broth. You can get several servings of dark leafy greens in just one bowl. The cashew cream and potato give the soup its heft and creaminess. A few air-fried croutons on top make a lovely textural contrast. This soup pairs well with Technicolor Tabbouleh Salad (page 97) or Baked Sweet Potatoes with Easy, Tasty Toppings (page 186).

Make the cashew cream. Soak the cashews in water for 2 hours or pour boiling water over them, cover, let them soak for about 20 minutes, then drain them. Set aside.

¼ cup raw cashews

Put them in a small blender with the water. Blend on high for 30 seconds or longer, until the cashews are dissolved. Set aside.

½ cup water

Make the soup. In a Dutch oven or soup pot, water sauté the onions and garlic until the onions are tender and transparent, 8 to 10 minutes.

1 medium red, yellow, or white onion, diced (about 1½ cups)
2 cloves garlic, finely chopped

Add in the following ingredients, bring the soup to a boil, then turn the heat down and simmer, partially covered, for about 10 minutes until the potatoes are tender.

4 cups vegetable broth
1 russet potato, peeled and chopped into chunks
1 bunch green onions, sliced

Add in the following ingredients and cook a few minutes more until the spinach is soft and still bright green.

The cashew cream
16 ounces fresh spinach (trim off thick stems if you are using mature, rather than baby, spinach)

Once the spinach is tender and bright green, add in the following ingredients and use a stick (immersion) blender to blend the soup into a puree.

(Continued on next page)

1 tablespoon nutritional yeast

2 teaspoons yellow or white miso

2 teaspoons freshly squeezed lemon juice

Optional spices: 1 teaspoon cumin or 1 teaspoon dill weed or 1 teaspoon curry powder

Salt and pepper to taste

The soup is ready to serve. Garnish each bowl of soup, if desired, with one or more of the following toppings.

Vegan crema or sour cream

Croutons

Pepitas

Roasted cumin seeds

This soup will last about a week in the refrigerator. It freezes well.

Moroccan Chickpea Soup

Makes 9 servings

This wonderfully complex soup used to take me over twenty-four hours to make, including soaking time. Now I make it in ninety minutes, start to finish, with an electric pressure cooker. I call this an "everything soup" because it contains beans, lentils, whole grain pasta, and vegetables. The Moroccan spice combination gives this dish a North African cinnamon-tinged vibe. This soup pairs well with Apple and Greens with Candied Walnuts (page 89) or Spinach and Apple Salad with Curry Dressing (page 86).

Pressure cooker directions. Add the following ingredients to an electric pressure cooker. Lock the lid. Move the knob to "Sealing." Use the "Manual," "Pressure Cook," or "High" mode and set for 35 minutes. When the pressure cooker is done, immediately move the knob to "Venting" and release the remaining steam before opening the lid.

> **7 cups water**
> **1½ cups dried chickpeas**

After opening the lid, add the following ingredients. Reseal the lid, move the knob to "Sealing," use the "Manual," "Pressure Cook," or "High" mode and set for 10 minutes. When the pressure cooker is done, immediately move the knob to "Venting" and release the remaining steam before opening the lid.

> **1 large red, yellow, or white onion, diced (about 2 cups)**
> **1 large celery stalk and leaves, finely chopped**
> **1 (28-ounce) can crushed tomatoes**
> **1 cup uncooked brown lentils**
> **⅓ cup fresh cilantro, chopped**
> **1 teaspoon turmeric**
> **½ teaspoon cinnamon**
> **Freshly ground black pepper to taste**

After opening the lid, stir in the pasta, then close the lid, leave the pressure cooker on low, and let the soup sit for about 10 minutes. Then, open the lid and stir—the pasta will be cooked.

> **2 ounces uncooked whole wheat angel hair or thin spaghetti, broken into 1" pieces (about ¾ cup)**

Finally, stir in the following ingredients.

> **½ cup fresh parsley, chopped**

(Continued on page 117)

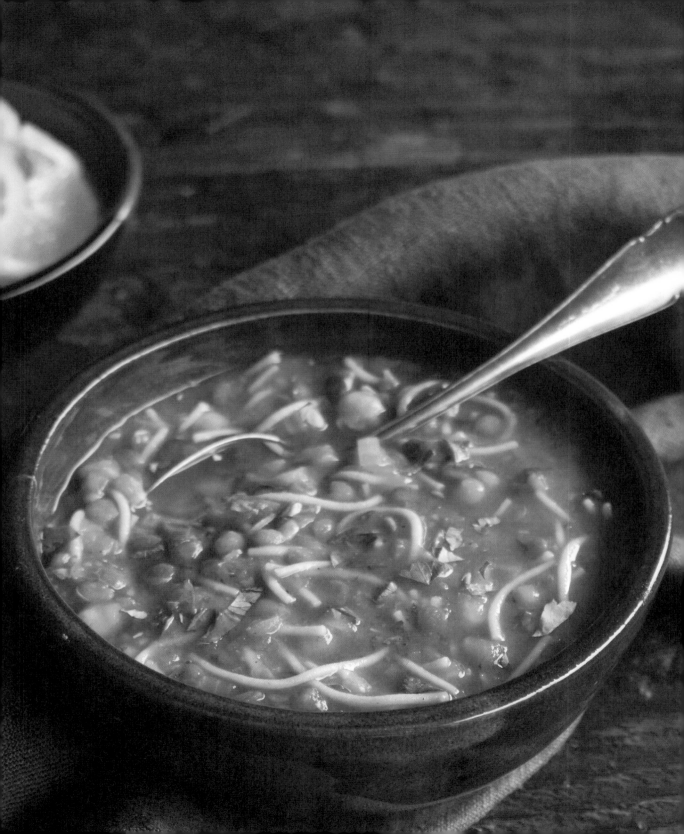

⅓ cup fresh cilantro, chopped

1¼ teaspoons salt (or to taste)

Stovetop directions (with canned chickpeas). Water sauté the onion and celery in a soup pot or Dutch oven until the onion is tender and transparent, 8 to 10 minutes. Add the crushed tomatoes, lentils, cilantro, turmeric, cinnamon, black pepper, 5 cups vegetable broth, and 3 (15-ounce) cans chickpeas, drained and rinsed. Stir to combine everything, raise the heat to bring the mixture to a boil, then turn the heat to low. Cover with the lid slightly ajar and let simmer for 45 minutes or until the lentils are fully tender (add more broth as needed). Stir in the angel hair or spaghetti and cook, uncovered, for 10 to 12 minutes until the pasta is tender. Finally, stir in the parsley, additional cilantro, and salt.

The soup is ready to eat. Serve with lemon wedges for those who want to squeeze them over their soup before eating.

Lemon wedges

The soup will keep at least a week in the refrigerator and can also be frozen.

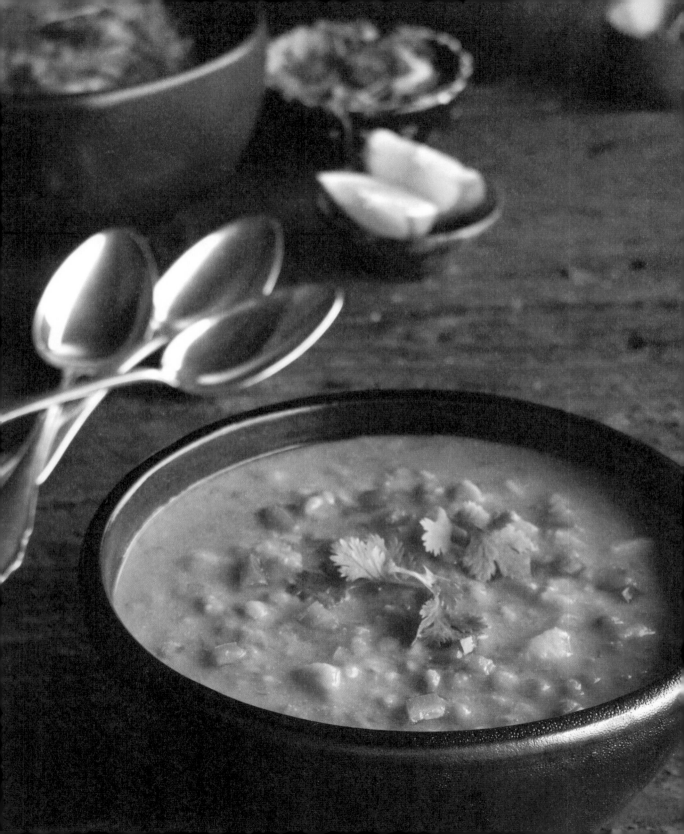

Thai-Inspired Creamy Sweet Potato and Lentil Soup

Makes 7 servings

Love lentil soup but want a variation? Studded with chunks of sweet potato and red bell pepper and spiced with curry paste, ginger, and lime, this soup will give you just the change of pace you're looking for. It's easy to make in a pressure cooker or on the stove. You could use any winter squash instead of the sweet potatoes and tomatoes instead of the bell pepper. I like this soup with Black Bean Burgers (page 197) or Curried Amaranth Patties (page 161) on whole grain bread or buns.

Soak the cashews. Soak the cashews in water for 2 hours or pour boiling water over them, cover, let them soak for about 20 minutes, then drain them. Set aside.

3 tablespoons raw cashews

Start the soup. Add the following ingredients to an electric pressure cooker. Lock the lid. Move the knob to "Sealing." Use the "Manual," "Pressure Cook," or "High" mode and set for 10 minutes.

6 cups vegetable broth
1 small red, yellow, or white onion, diced (about 1 cup)
1 (12-ounce) medium sweet potato, peeled, cut into ½-inch pieces
1½ cups uncooked brown or red lentils
1 medium or large red bell pepper, diced
2 teaspoons fresh ginger, finely chopped

Make the cashew mixture. While the soup is cooking, put the following ingredients in a blender. Blend on high for 30 seconds or longer, until the cashews are dissolved. Set aside.

The soaked and drained cashews
1 cup water
2½ tablespoons soy sauce or tamari
Juice from 1 lime (1½ tablespoons)
1 tablespoon Thai curry paste, red curry paste, Massaman paste, or yellow curry paste (see box on page 120 for more about Thai curry pastes)
2 Medjool dates, cut into a few pieces

(Continued on next page)

Finish the soup. Wait for 10 minutes once the pressure cooker is done, then move the knob to "Venting" and release the remaining steam before opening the lid. Add the following ingredients to the pressure cooker. Stir for a couple of minutes to allow the cashew mixture to thicken.

The cashew mixture
¼ cup fresh cilantro, chopped

Stovetop directions. Increase the vegetable broth to 7 cups. Combine the first set of ingredients in a soup pot or Dutch oven. Bring to a boil, then lower the heat and simmer, covered or partially covered, until the lentils are done and the sweet potatoes are tender, about 45 minutes. Once everything is tender, add the cashew mixture and cilantro and cook on low for a few minutes to allow the cashew mixture to thicken.

Salt will likely not be needed because of the soy sauce but add in salt if desired and adjust any other seasonings.

Salt to taste

Garnish with additional cilantro if desired.

This soup is ready to serve. It will keep for about a week in the refrigerator. It can also be frozen.

Thai curry pastes are mixtures of pulverized chilis, herbs, and spices. Many people make their own, but most of us use canned curry pastes. The blends of chilis, garlic, shallots, lemongrass, galangal, cilantro, and other ingredients create irresistible aromas and flavors in soups, stews, curries, and other dishes. There are five common types of curry paste:

- Red (spicy)—is considered the "default" curry paste.
- Green (very spicy)—uses similar ingredients to red curry paste but calls for fresh green chilis instead of dried red chilis.
- Panang (spicy)—is similar to red but includes roasted peanuts and additional spices like cumin and coriander.
- Massaman (medium spicy)—uses fragrant spices like cardamom, nutmeg, and cloves.
- Yellow (mildly spicy)—gets its color from turmeric and curry powder.

Read the labels to make sure your curry paste is vegan. Once you open a can, you can use part of it and freeze the rest for later use.

Black Bean and Rice Soup

Makes 7 servings

This soup epitomizes the saying, "The whole is greater than the sum of its parts." The ingredients number fewer than ten, but the final result tastes much more complex than that. Plus, the soup is low in fat and high in fiber. A single batch could easily provide a week's worth of lunches if you're so inclined, or you can put some in the freezer. It goes well with Spicy Sweet Potato Chipotle Quesadillas with Guacamole (page 189) and a salad for a filling dinner.

Add the following ingredients to an electric pressure cooker. Lock the lid. Move the knob to "Sealing." Use the "Manual," "Pressure Cook," or "High" mode and set for 24 minutes.

> **8½ cups water**
> **1 pound (about 2½ cups) uncooked black beans**
> **½ cup uncooked brown rice, rinsed**
> **1 medium red, yellow, or white onion, diced (about 1½ cups)**
> **5 cloves garlic, finely chopped**
> **1 tablespoon chili powder**
> **1½ teaspoons cumin**
> **1½ teaspoons oregano or Mexican oregano**
> **1 teaspoon smoked paprika**

Wait for 10 to 20 minutes once the pressure cooker is done, then move the knob to "Venting" and release the remaining steam before opening the lid. Add the following ingredients to the pressure cooker.

> **2 tablespoons red wine vinegar**
> **1½ teaspoons salt (or to taste)**

Use a stick (immersion) blender or a potato masher to blend some of the soup for a creamier texture, leaving most of the beans whole. Taste and add more vinegar or salt as desired.

Stovetop directions. Increase the water to 9 cups. Soak the black beans overnight, then drain and rinse them. Put everything except the vinegar and salt in a soup pot or Dutch oven. Bring to a boil, reduce heat to a low simmer, cover the pot, and start checking for doneness after 45 minutes. It may take 30 or 45 minutes longer than that, depending on your beans, water, and heat. When done, add in the vinegar and salt and blend as described above.

(Continued on page 123)

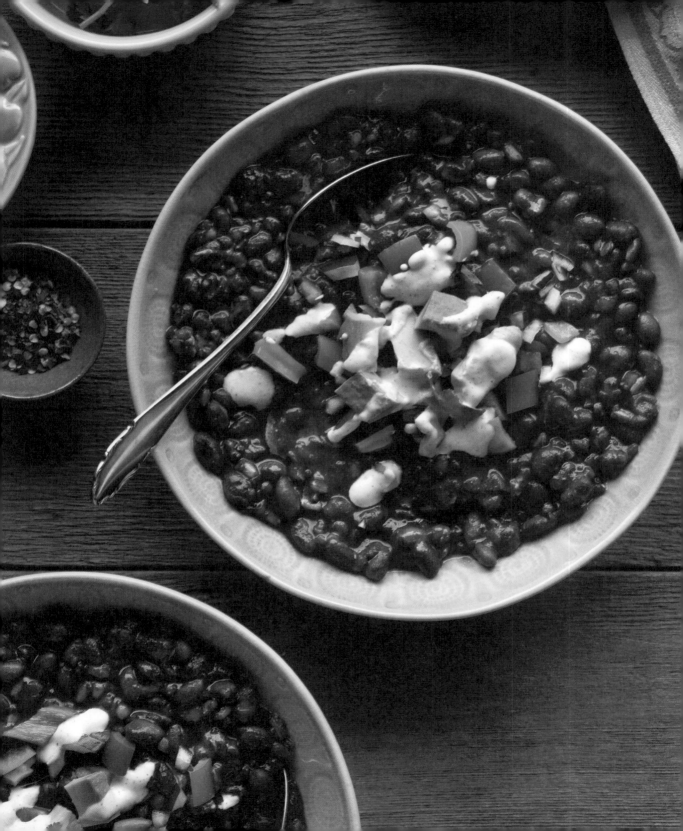

This soup is ready to serve. Garnish each bowl, if desired, with one or more of the following toppings.

Vegan crema or sour cream
Sliced green onions
Sliced radishes
Chopped tomatoes
Finely chopped red bell peppers

The soup will last about a week in the refrigerator and freezes well.

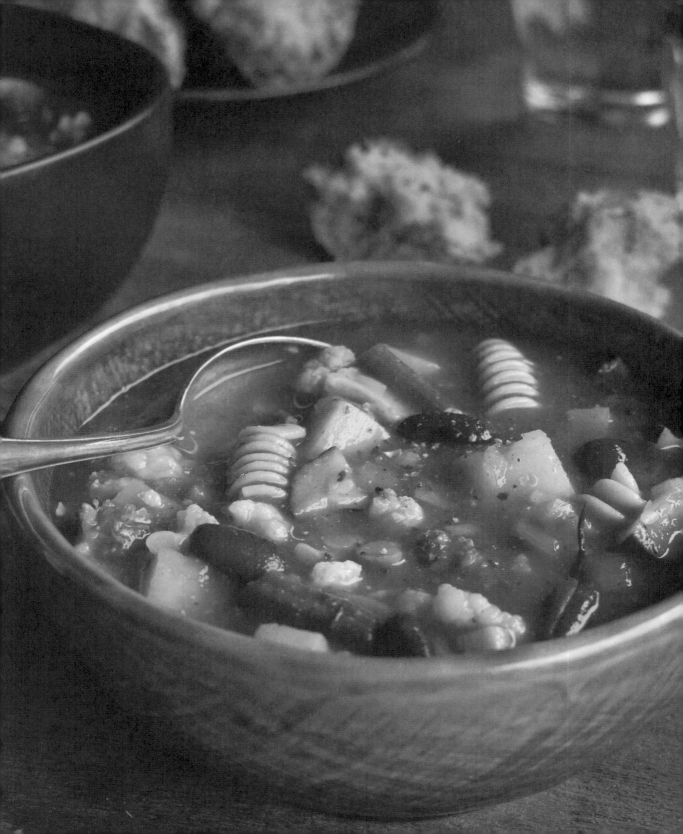

Minestrone Soup with Kidney or Red Beans

Makes 5 servings

Research has shown that starting a meal with a light vegetable soup leads to fewer total calories consumed. This is the perfect soup for that purpose. With its brothy texture, it also serves as an excellent lunchtime soup on its own or in a soup-and-salad or soup-and-sandwich combination. The vegetable combination is flexible, so make it your way and use any pasta shapes that make you smile.

Water sauté the onion and garlic in a Dutch oven or soup pot until the onion is tender and transparent, 8 to 10 minutes.

1 medium red, yellow, or white onion, diced (about 1½ cups)
2 cloves garlic, finely chopped

Add the following ingredients, bring to a boil, then reduce the heat and simmer on low, partially covered, for 20 minutes, stirring occasionally.

1 (15-ounce) can crushed tomatoes or tomato sauce
1 (15-ounce) can kidney beans or small red beans, drained and rinsed
4 cups vegetable broth
2 cups zucchini, broccoli, green beans, and/or cauliflower, small-diced
1 large carrot, peeled and diced
1 large celery stalk or several small ones, sliced or diced
1 red or Yukon potato, diced (peeling is optional)
1 teaspoon basil
1 teaspoon thyme
1 teaspoon salt (or to taste)
½ teaspoon dried oregano
Freshly ground black pepper to taste

Add pasta, partially cover, and cook an additional 10 minutes or longer if the pasta needs more time.

¼ cup uncooked pasta, e.g., whole wheat elbow macaroni, broken spaghetti, shells

Adjust spices to suit your taste. The soup is ready to serve.

This soup will last about a week in the refrigerator and freezes well.

Yellow Curry Soup with Black Rice

Makes 6 servings

Black rice is also called "forbidden rice" or "emperor's rice" because it was once reserved for the Chinese emperor and aristocracy. It's come a long way—I can buy it in a grocery store bulk section today! It has a nutty flavor similar to wild rice and is packed with anti-inflammatory anthocyanins, which give it its blackish-purple color. Here it's used in a fragrant soup flavored with yellow curry paste. Since this soup is almost a meal in itself, it pairs well with a light salad like Grapefruit and Avocado Salad (page 85).

Make cashew milk. Soak the cashews in water for 2 hours or pour boiling water over them, cover, let them soak for about 20 minutes, then drain them. Set aside.

> ⅓ **cup raw cashews**

Put them in a blender with the water. Blend on high for 30 seconds or longer, until the cashews are dissolved. Set aside.

> 1½ **cups water**

Make the black rice. Cook the rice according to the Whole Grains Cooking Guide on page 43.

> 1½ **cups uncooked black rice**
> 3 **cups water for stovetop or** 1¾ **cups water for pressure cooker**

Make the soup. In a Dutch oven or soup pot, water sauté the following ingredients until the onions are tender and transparent, 8 to 10 minutes.

> 1 **medium red, yellow, or white onion, diced (about** 1½ **cups)**
> 2 **medium carrots, peeled and diced**
> 2 **cloves garlic, finely chopped**

Add in the following ingredients, bring to a boil, then reduce the heat and simmer on low, uncovered, for 8 to 10 minutes, stirring occasionally until the bell pepper and sweet potato are tender.

> 1 **red bell pepper, diced**
> 1 **medium sweet potato, peeled and diced into** ½-**inch cubes**
> 3 **cups vegetable stock**
> 2 **tablespoons yellow curry paste (see box on page 120 for more about Thai curry pastes)**
> 1 **tablespoon soy sauce or tamari**

(Continued on page 128)

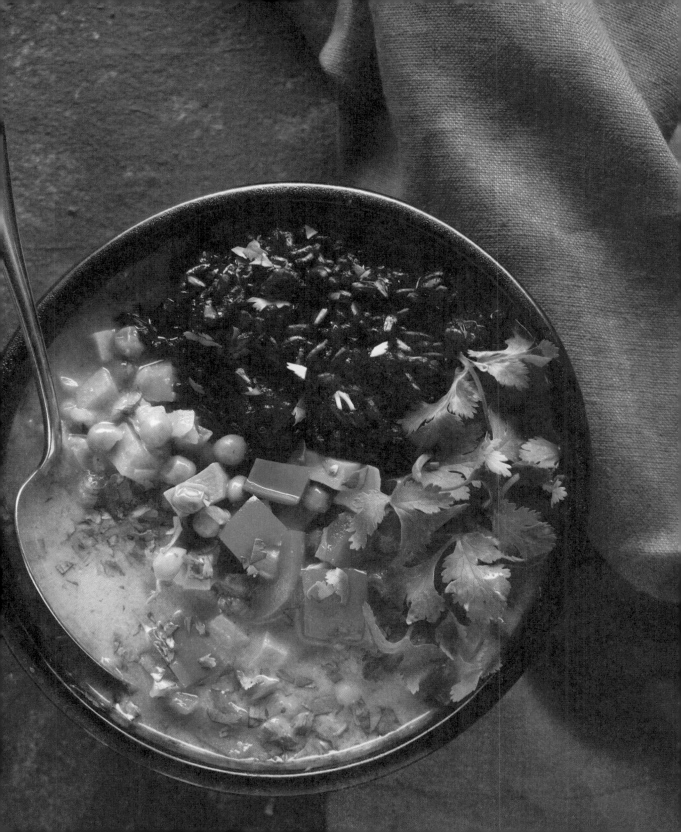

½ teaspoon turmeric
Zest from ½ lime

Add the following ingredients and bring the mixture to a boil, then turn down the heat and allow to simmer, uncovered, for about 4 minutes, stirring often to prevent the cashew milk from burning on the bottom of the pan.

The cashew milk
1 cup frozen peas

Stir in the following ingredients and remove the soup from the heat. Taste and adjust lime juice, salt, and/or curry paste.

2 green onions, sliced
2–3 tablespoons fresh cilantro, chopped
1–2 tablespoons fresh lime juice
1 teaspoon salt (or to taste)

The soup is ready to serve. Spoon a scoop of black rice into each bowl, then ladle the soup around it and garnish with the following ingredients if desired.

Sliced green onions
Chopped fresh cilantro
Finely diced red bell pepper or chilis

The soup lasts for about a week in the refrigerator and can be frozen. Store the rice and soup separately.

Massaman Peanut Noodle Soup

Makes 4 servings

This mouthwatering soup features peanuts, noodles, and a creamy broth. You'd have had me at peanuts, but the combination of these three elements, plus hints of lime and curry paste to jazz things up, makes for a full-bodied flavor and texture that always satisfies. Instead of millet and brown rice ramen, you could also try buckwheat soba noodles or even whole wheat angel hair pasta. This soup pairs well with Fruit Salad with a Hint of Ginger (page 81).

Make the peanut butter broth. Blend together the following ingredients on high for 30 seconds or longer, until the dates are dissolved. Set the broth aside.

2½ cups vegetable broth
⅓ cup natural peanut butter (creamy or chunky)
3 Medjool dates, each cut into a few pieces

Make the soup. In a Dutch oven or soup pot, broth sauté the vegetables (start with ¼ cup vegetable broth) for 8 to 10 minutes, until the sweet potato is just tender.

1 medium sweet potato, peeled and diced
1 red bell pepper, diced

Combine the following ingredients in the pot and cook for another few minutes on medium, stirring frequently.

1 clove garlic, finely chopped
1 tablespoon fresh ginger, finely chopped
1–2 tablespoons Massaman curry paste, yellow curry paste, or red curry paste (see box on
**   page 120 for more about Thai curry pastes)**
¾ teaspoon smoked paprika
½ teaspoon turmeric

Increase the heat, add in the following ingredients, and bring to a low boil. Cook, uncovered, stirring often for about 5 minutes, until the thickness is to your liking.

The peanut butter broth
3 cups vegetable broth
Juice from 1 lime (1–2 tablespoons)
2 tablespoons soy sauce or tamari
1 teaspoon Chinese roasted sesame paste (see box page 131) or sesame oil

Add in the noodles and cook for 3 minutes.

(Continued on page 131)

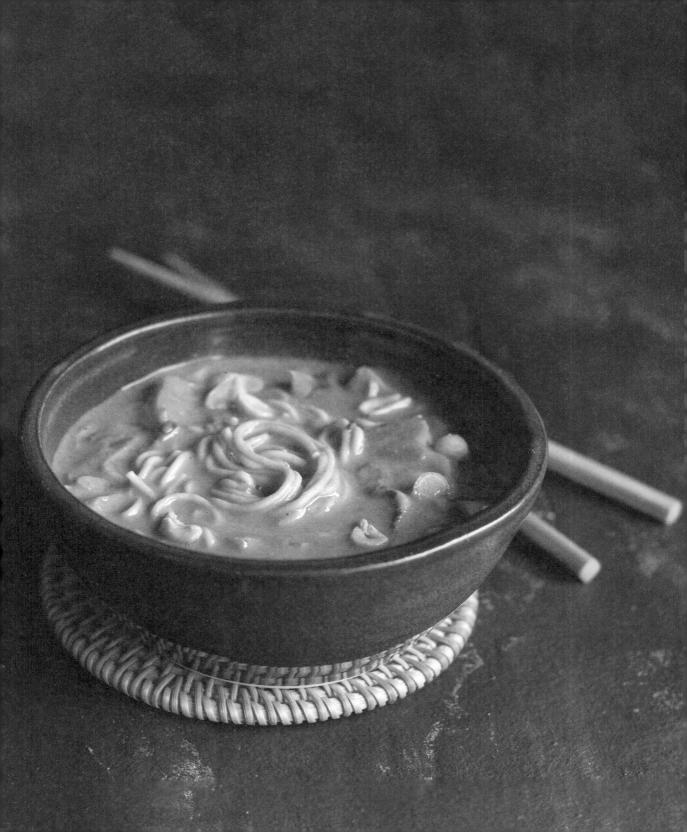

3 ounces whole grain thin noodles (millet and brown rice ramen noodles recommended)

To serve, ladle soup into bowls and divide the following garnishes among the bowls.

4 green onions, thinly sliced
¼ cup chopped peanuts
¼ cup chopped fresh cilantro

This soup will last about a week in the refrigerator. It does not freeze well. The noodles will absorb more of the broth, so you may need to add more water if reheating.

Chinese roasted sesame paste

This paste is the key ingredient in cold sesame noodles, a favorite appetizer in many Chinese restaurants in the United States, but it's also a fantastic whole-food replacement for sesame oil in all sorts of recipes. It's a thick, dark brown paste made from ground roasted sesame seeds. Tahini is also made from ground sesame seeds, but the seeds are not roasted as long as those used in Chinese roasted sesame paste. The latter smells and tastes more like sesame oil than tahini does. You can find roasted sesame paste in most Asian grocery stores or online.

Tomato and Roasted Red Pepper Soup

Makes 4 servings

Adding roasted red peppers to a basic tomato soup increases the complexity of the flavor and provides an appetizing orange hue. Cashews provide extra creaminess here, and simple spices deepen the flavors. For a meal in a bowl, you could add cooked greens (spinach, chard, kale), cooked beans, and/or baked tofu or grated tempeh for extra antioxidants, protein, and fiber. I like this soup with whole grain bread and a salad such as the Lemony Farro and Bean Salad (page 103).

Soak the cashews in water for 2 hours or pour boiling water over them, cover, let them soak for about 20 minutes, then drain them.

½ cup raw cashews

Put the cashews in a blender with the water. Blend on high for 30 seconds or longer, until the cashews are dissolved.

2 cups water

Put the remaining ingredients in the blender and blend until smooth.

1 cup vegetable broth
1 cup roasted red bell peppers (if from a jar, rinsed)
¾ cup (6 ounces) tomato paste
2 teaspoons onion powder
1 teaspoon salt (or to taste)
½ teaspoon oregano
¼ teaspoon garlic powder
Freshly ground black pepper to taste

Put the soup in a Dutch oven or soup pot, bring to a boil, lower, and simmer for about 5 minutes until thickened. The soup is ready to serve. It will last in the refrigerator for 4 to 5 days and freezes well.

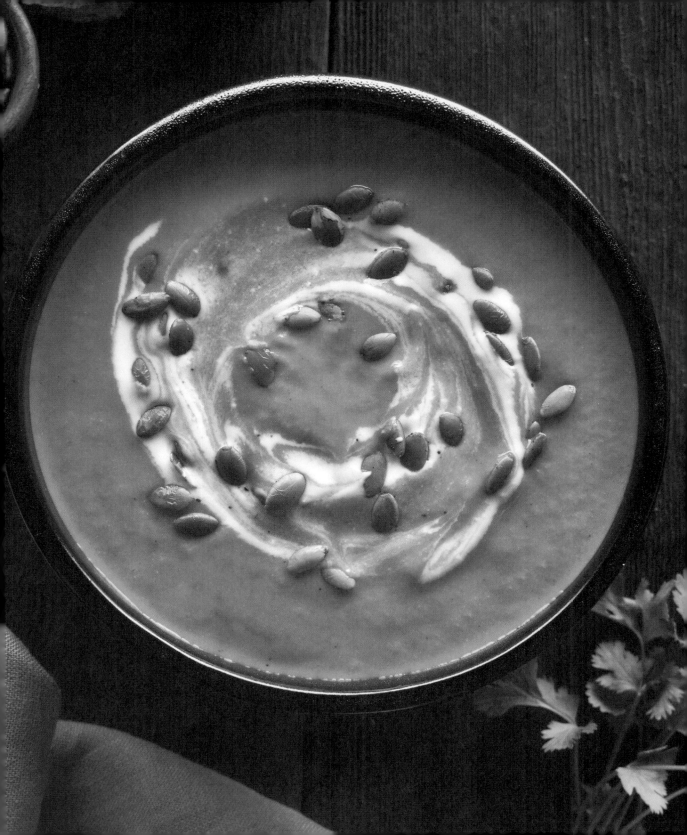

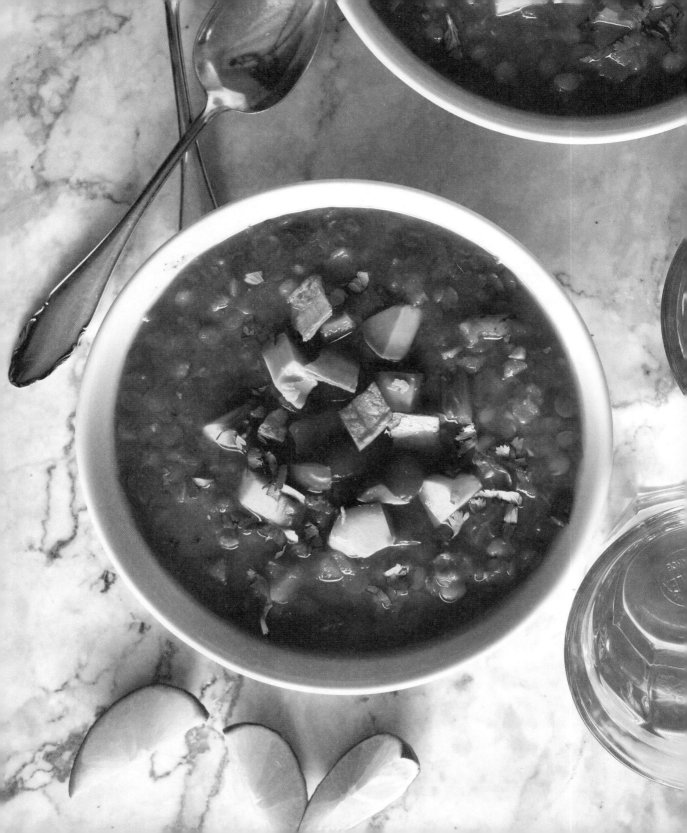

Mexican-Inspired Lentil Soup

Makes 6 servings

I've coached a lot of students in plant-based eating and cooking, and I can't think of a single one of them who didn't like lentil soup. For their sake I've tried to create variations on lentil soup over the years to increase the number of ways they can eat this superbly healthy legume. Lentils and Mexican spices go very well together, perhaps because lentils have an earthy flavor similar to pinto beans. This soup pairs nicely with Spicy Sweet Potato Chipotle Quesadillas with Guacamole (page 189).

Pressure cooker directions. Add the following ingredients to an electric pressure cooker. Lock the lid. Move the valve to "Sealing." Use the "Manual," "Pressure Cook," or "High" mode and set for 10 minutes. Wait for 10 minutes after the pressure cooker is done, then move the knob to "Venting" and release the remaining steam before opening the lid.

6 cups vegetable broth
1 (15-ounce) can petite diced or diced tomatoes (fire-roasted, if available)
1 (4-ounce) can mild green chiles, undrained
1¼ cups uncooked brown lentils
1 medium red, yellow, or white onion, diced (about 1½ cups)
2 celery stalks, diced
2 medium carrots, diced
4 cloves garlic, finely chopped
2 bay leaves
1 tablespoon chili powder, chipotle powder, or ancho chili powder
2 teaspoons cumin
½ teaspoon oregano
½ teaspoon coriander
½ teaspoon smoked paprika

After opening the pressure cooker, add the following ingredients and stir to combine. Adjust seasonings (more lime, cilantro, chili powder, salt) and serve.

¼ cup fresh cilantro, chopped
2 teaspoons lime juice (or more to taste)
1 teaspoon salt (or to taste)
Freshly ground black pepper to taste

If you want a creamier soup, pulse it a few times with a stick (immersion) blender.

(Continued on next page)

Stovetop directions. In a soup pot or Dutch oven, increase the water to 6½ cups. Combine all remaining ingredients above except the cilantro, lime juice, salt, and pepper. Bring to a boil, reduce heat to a low simmer, cover the pot all the way or partway, and simmer for 45 minutes. When done, add in the cilantro, lime juice, salt, and pepper.

The soup is ready to serve. Garnish, if desired, with one or more of the following toppings.

Chopped fresh cilantro
Sliced avocado
Sliced green onions
Sliced jalapeños

This soup will keep in the refrigerator for about a week. It freezes well.

The Plant-Based Anti-Inflammatory Cookbook

White Bean Soup with Rosemary

Makes 6 servings

One of the perks of moving from the East Coast to Oregon is being able to grow rosemary plants and use their fresh leaves all year round, since rosemary loves the dry heat of Western summers. As an anti-inflammatory superstar, rosemary shines in this simple but flavorful recipe. Cannellini beans are my favorite white beans because of their creaminess, but navy and Great Northern beans also work well in this dish. With hearty bread and Apple and Greens with Candied Walnuts (page 89), this soup makes a fine dinner.

Pressure cooker directions. Add the following ingredients to an electric pressure cooker. Lock the lid. Move the knob to "Sealing." Use the "Manual," "High," or "Pressure Cook" mode and set for 25 minutes for navy beans, 30 minutes for cannellini beans, or 40 minutes for Great Northern beans. Wait 15 to 20 minutes after the pressure cooker is done, then move the knob to "Venting" and release the remaining steam before opening the lid. Check the beans' texture. If they are not soft enough, put the lid back on and set for 5 minutes on the same settings.

> 1 pound (about 2½ cups) dried navy, cannellini, or Great Northern beans, unsoaked
> 7½ cups water
> 4 cloves garlic, finely chopped
> 4 teaspoons fresh chopped rosemary or 1½ teaspoons dried rosemary, crushed
> 2 teaspoons thyme
> 2 teaspoons oregano

After opening the pressure cooker, add the following ingredients and stir to combine.

> 4 teaspoons sherry vinegar, champagne vinegar, or white wine vinegar (see box on page 88)
> 1 teaspoon salt (or to taste)
> Freshly ground black pepper to taste

If desired, use a stick (immersion) blender or a potato masher to create a creamier soup. I like to leave it a bit chunky rather than completely smooth. You may need to add water.

Stovetop directions with canned beans. Decrease the water to 5 cups. Use 4 (15-ounce) cans of cooked beans (drained and rinsed). Put all ingredients except the vinegar together in a soup pot or Dutch oven. Bring to a boil, reduce heat to a low simmer and cook, partially covered, for about 20 minutes, stirring every 5 minutes or so (because the beans can burn on the bottom of the pans). Once you have the texture you desire, stir in the vinegar and follow the final directions above.

(Continued on page 139)

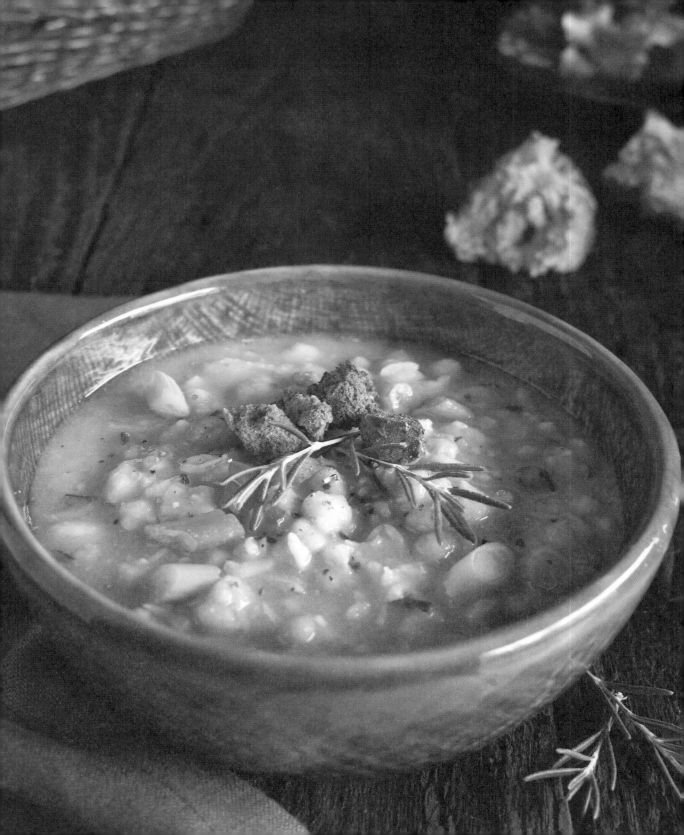

The soup is ready to serve. Garnish each bowl of soup, if desired, with one or more of the following toppings.

Sliced green onions
Croutons
Vegan Parmesan
Chopped sun-dried tomatoes

This soup keeps in the refrigerator for about a week. It also freezes well.

Creamy Wild Rice and Mushroom Soup

Makes 6 servings

Fun fact: wild rice isn't rice. It's actually a grass that grows in water with grains that look, feel, and taste like rice. A few cashews give this soup a creaminess that takes it from good to great. I never get tired of this soup because the texture is so interesting—with the split wild rice, chewy mushrooms, and tender vegetables—and the taste—it's an umami lover's delight. This soup pairs well with potatoes, any roasted or steamed vegetable, whole grain bread, and/ or a light salad.

Make the cashew milk. Soak the cashews in water for 2 hours or pour boiling water over them, cover, let them soak for about 20 minutes, then drain them.

½ cup raw cashews

Put them in a blender with the water. Blend on high for 30 seconds or longer, until the cashews are dissolved.

1½ cups water

Pressure cooker directions. Add the following ingredients to an electric pressure cooker. Lock the lid. Move the knob to "Sealing." Use the "Manual," "Pressure Cook," or "High" mode and set for 30 minutes.

½ medium red, yellow, or white onion, diced (about ¾ cup)
8 ounces fresh cremini and/or white button mushrooms, sliced, diced, or chopped
5 cups vegetable broth
¾ cup uncooked wild rice, rinsed
⅓ cup uncooked brown lentils
2 teaspoons thyme
1 teaspoon oregano
1 teaspoon sage
1 teaspoon salt (or to taste)

When the pressure cooker is done, immediately move the knob to "Venting" and release the remaining steam before opening the lid. Add the following ingredients, then relock the lid, move the knob to "Sealing," use the "Manual," "Pressure Cook," or "High" mode and set for 8 minutes.

(Continued on page 142)

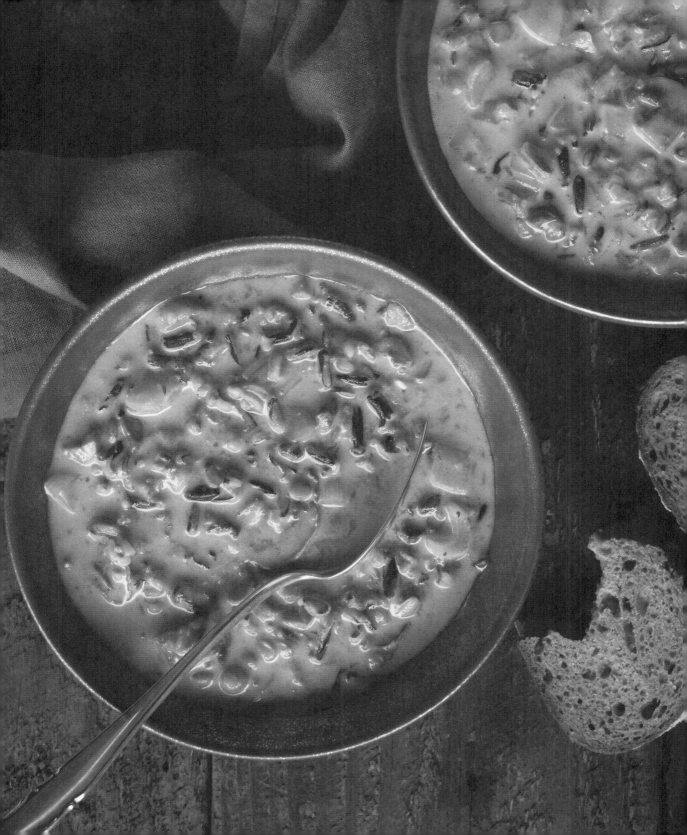

3 cloves garlic, finely chopped
2 medium or large carrots, diced
3 celery stalks, diced

When the pressure cooker is done, immediately move the knob to "Venting" and release the remaining steam before opening the lid.

Add the following ingredients and stir the soup continuously to heat up the cashew milk and get it to thicken. If needed, turn the pressure cooker to "Sauté" mode to boil the mixture. After 2 to 3 minutes of stirring and/or boiling, the cashew milk should be adequately cooked.

The cashew milk
1 tablespoon Braggs Liquid Aminos, 2 teaspoons soy sauce (or tamari), or 1 teaspoon umami mushroom seasoning

Taste and add more seasonings and/or water as needed.

Stovetop directions. Make the cashew milk as indicated above. Water sauté the onions and mushrooms in a Dutch oven or soup pot until the onions are tender and transparent, 8 to 10 minutes. Then, add in the vegetable broth (increase to 5½ cups), wild rice, lentils, thyme, oregano, sage, and salt. Bring to a boil, then reduce to a simmer, cover, and cook for 40 minutes. Add in the garlic, carrots, and celery and bring to a simmer again. Cover, and cook for 10 minutes more until the carrots and celery are tender. Add in the remaining ingredients and bring to a gentle boil, stirring frequently, uncovered, for 3 to 4 minutes so that the cashew milk thickens the soup. Add more water if needed. Taste and adjust seasonings.

This soup is ready to serve. It will keep well for about a week in the refrigerator—you may need to add more water or nondairy milk to thin it out. It can be frozen.

The Plant-Based Anti-Inflammatory Cookbook

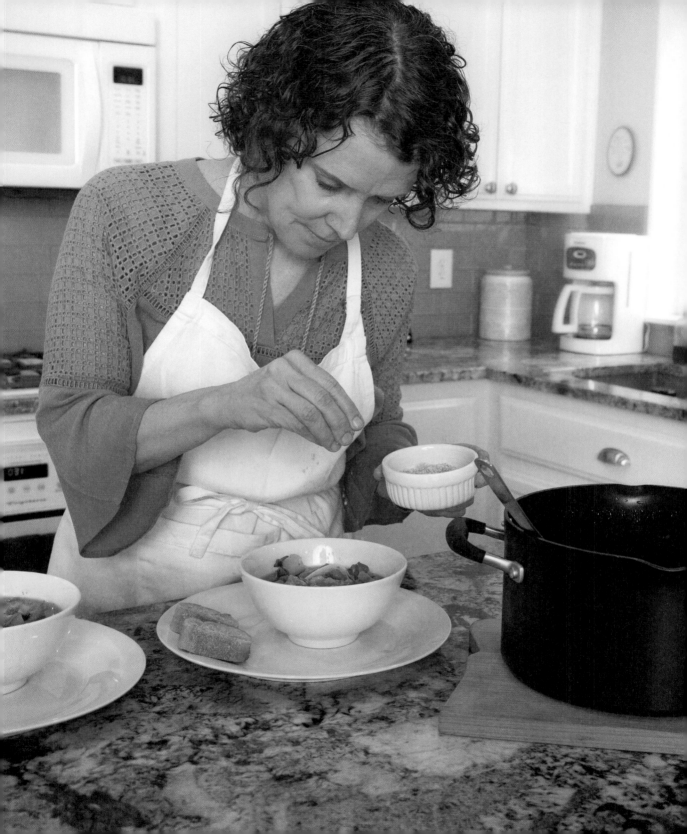

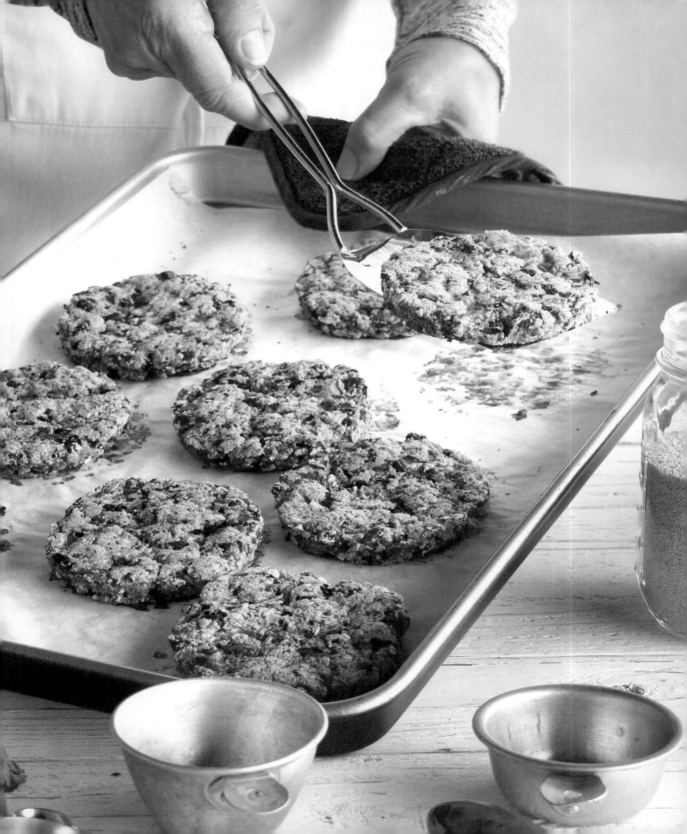

Whole Grains

Grains . . . carbs . . . the enemy? No! Whole grains provide healthy fuel for muscles and brains. As part of a healthy, anti-inflammatory approach to eating, whole grains contribute valuable fiber and slow-digesting carbohydrates. This prevents a post-meal sugar rush and free-radical surge and feeds the good gut bacteria that produce inflammation calming, short-chain fatty acids.

So many grains, so little time. The possibilities are endless with grains and pseudo-grains like quinoa, rice, polenta, millet, freekeh, farro, amaranth, and others. I hope you find these recipes to be delicious on their own, but also starting points for your own take on tasty grain dishes. Grain salads usually last well in the refrigerator for several days, meaning delicious leftovers on nights when you might not feel like cooking.

Check out my Whole Grains Cooking Guide (page 43) for the basics on cooking up whole grains on the stove or in a pressure cooker. That's where the magic begins.

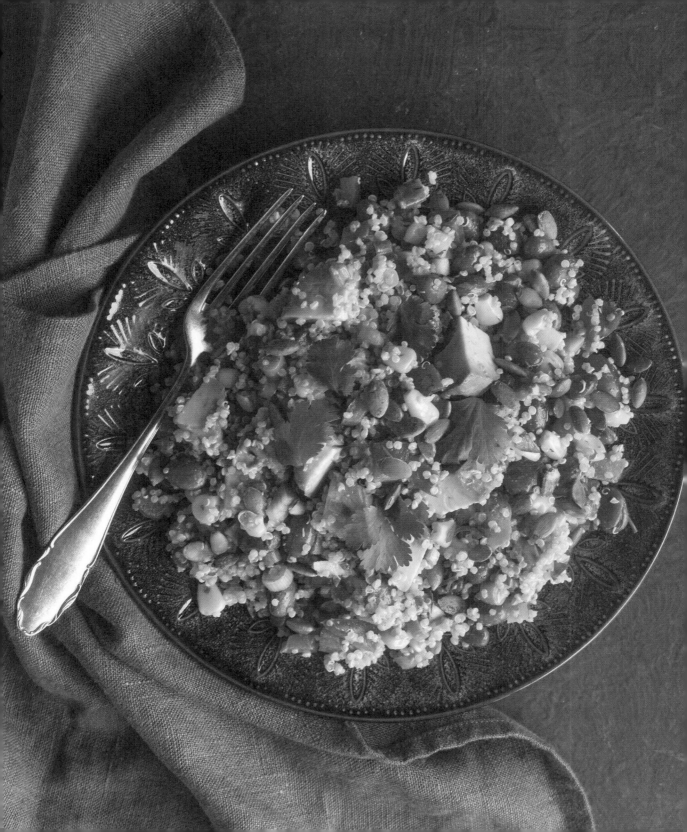

Kaleidoscopic Quinoa Salad

Makes 6 servings

Many of my students love having a healthy salad in their fridge for quick lunches. (So do I!) This is one of those salads that lasts almost a week without spoiling or wilting. High in protein and anti-inflammatory compounds, this dish lets you "eat the rainbow" and increase the diversity of plants in your diet. You can switch out any of the vegetables or beans. The salad goes well with a creamy soup or Black Bean Burgers (page 197).

Make the dressing. Whisk the following ingredients together in a bowl or blend them in a small blender. Set aside.

- ¼ cup freshly squeezed lemon juice
- 2 tablespoons tahini
- 4 teaspoons red wine vinegar, white wine vinegar, sherry vinegar, or champagne vinegar (see box on page 88)
- ½ teaspoon cumin
- ½ teaspoon garlic powder
- ½ teaspoon salt (or to taste)
- Freshly ground pepper to taste

Make the salad. In a large mixing bowl or salad bowl, add the following ingredients and stir them until well incorporated.

- 1 cup quinoa from 1 cup uncooked (see the Whole Grains Cooking Guide on page 43 for instructions)
- 1 red bell pepper, diced
- 1 (15-ounce) can small red, black, or kidney beans, drained and rinsed
- 1–1½ cups fresh tomatoes, diced, or cherry tomatoes, halved
- ½–1 cup red onion, diced, or green onions, sliced
- 1 cup fresh or frozen and thawed corn
- ½ cup fresh cilantro, chopped
- 2 cloves garlic, finely chopped
- Optional: ½–1 jalapeño pepper, deveined and deseeded if desired, finely chopped
- Optional: 1 avocado, peeled and diced
- Optional: Handful of pepitas or other roasted seeds

Toss the dressing with the salad. Taste and adjust seasonings (especially lemon juice, salt, and cumin). Serve the salad immediately or chill to serve later. It will last 4 to 5 days in the refrigerator. It does not freeze well.

Freekeh Salad
with Roasted Sweet Potatoes

Makes 4 large servings

Freekeh is a whole grain with many pluses, especially its nutty flavor and relatively quick cooking time. In this salad, which could serve as a main dish and would travel well for a summer picnic, freekeh is tossed together with roasted sweet potatoes, currants, lemon zest, and a light dressing. It can be eaten cold or at room temperature. You can switch it up and try it with your own choice of roasted vegetables and dried fruit. This salad also pairs well with a bean or lentil soup for dinner.

Roast the vegetables. Use the Roasting Vegetables without Oil method (see on page 171) to roast the sweet potatoes.

1 pound sweet potatoes

Cook the freekeh. Cook the freekeh according to the Whole Grains Cooking Guide (see on page 43).

½ cup uncooked freekeh

Make the dressing. Whisk or shake the following ingredients together in a small bowl or jar.

2 tablespoons freshly squeezed lemon juice
1 tablespoon water
1 tablespoon tahini
1 teaspoon Dijon mustard
Salt and pepper to taste

Toss it together. In a large mixing bowl or salad bowl, toss together the following ingredients.

The roasted sweet potatoes
The cooked freekeh
½ cup currants, black raisins, golden raisins, or other dried fruit
1–3 teaspoons lemon zest (optional)

Drizzle with most of the dressing and toss to coat. Taste and adjust seasonings. Just before serving, stir in herb(s) of choice and use more of the dressing, if needed (or save the dressing for leftovers).

1–3 tablespoons finely chopped mint and/or other herbs (optional)

This salad will last 3 to 4 days in the refrigerator. It does not freeze well.

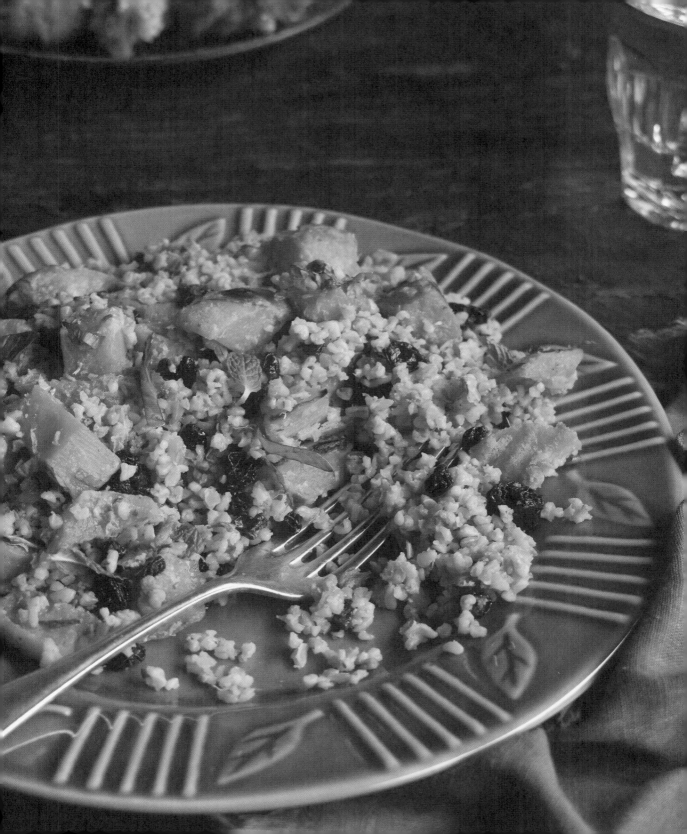

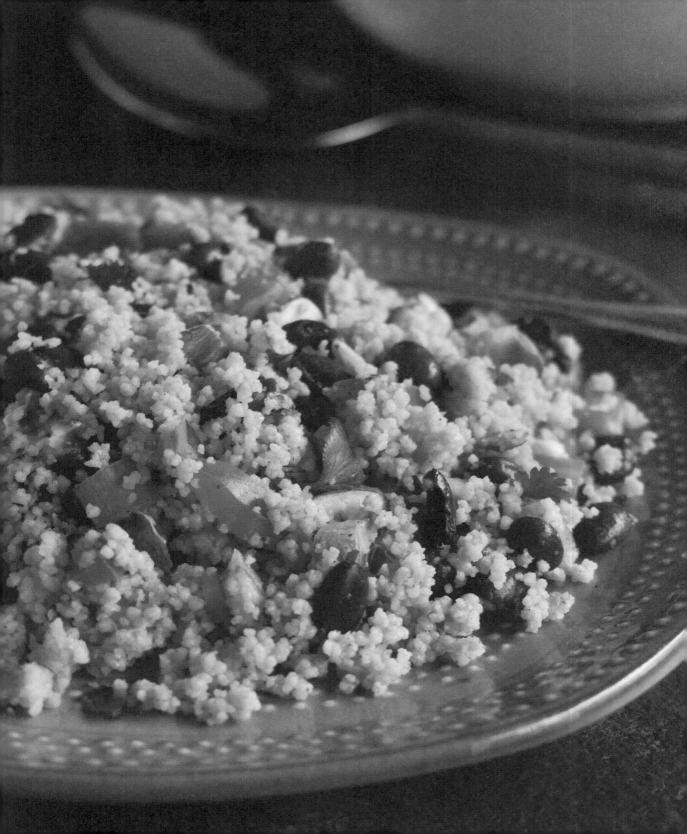

Orange-Infused Couscous Salad

Makes 6 servings

Couscous, a tiny pasta made from wheat flour, gets a double infusion of orange in this dish: from the orange juice and zest. The beans, vegetables, nuts, dried fruit, spices, and herbs transform the couscous into a lovely pilaf that pairs well with Curried Amaranth Patties (page 161), Savory Quinoa Cakes (page 164), or a bean soup.

Prep the oranges. Zest 1 orange and juice 2 oranges.

Zest from 1 navel orange
Juice from 2 navel oranges, divided

Make the couscous. In a small or medium saucepan, combine the following ingredients and bring to a boil.

¾ cup orange juice
½ cup water
1 teaspoon coriander
¼ teaspoon cinnamon
¼ teaspoon salt (or to taste)
Freshly ground black pepper to taste

Remove the saucepan from the heat and immediately stir in the couscous. Cover the pan and let it stand for 5 minutes, then fluff the couscous with a fork and cover again. Let it cool further, at least another 5 minutes.

1 cup uncooked whole wheat couscous

Toast the almonds. Add the almonds to a small skillet and cook them on medium heat for 3 minutes or until toasted, stirring or shaking frequently. Remove them from the pan as soon as they are toasted.

⅓ cup sliced or slivered almonds

Make the dressing. Whisk or shake the following ingredients together in a small bowl or jar.

The orange zest
The remaining orange juice
1 tablespoon freshly squeezed lime or lemon juice
1 tablespoon tahini

(Continued on next page)

2 teaspoons maple syrup

¼ teaspoon salt (or to taste)

Freshly ground black pepper to taste

Complete the salad. To a large mixing bowl or salad bowl, add the following ingredients and toss together.

The fluffed couscous

The toasted almonds

1 (15-ounce) can small red, kidney, or black beans, drained and rinsed

½ cup chopped or sliced celery (2 small stalks or 1 large)

½ cup chopped red bell pepper

¼ cup chopped red onion

¼ cup chopped fresh cilantro

¼ cup dried cherries, cranberries, or other dried fruit

Drizzle the dressing over the couscous mixture and toss to coat everything. Taste and adjust seasonings. The salad is ready to serve, but it will improve after 1 to 2 hours as the flavors blend. This salad will keep in the refrigerator for 3 to 4 days. It does not freeze well.

Rice Pilaf with Mushrooms and Pine Nuts

Makes about 5 cups

Broth, miso, and mushrooms give this pilaf its satisfying umami flavor. It pairs well as a side dish to many entrees, including shepherd's pie or Savory Quinoa Cakes (page 164) and gravy. It also adds depth and flavor to a bowl with roasted vegetables, beans or baked tofu, and a sauce or gravy.

Pressure cooker directions. Add the following ingredients to an electric pressure cooker. Lock the lid. Move the knob to "Sealing." Use the "Multigrain," "Manual," "Pressure Cook," or "High" mode and set for 21 minutes. Wait 10 minutes after the pressure cooker is done, then move the knob to "Venting" and release any remaining steam before opening the lid.

- 1½ cups uncooked brown rice, rinsed
- 2⅛ cups vegetable broth
- ¼ teaspoon salt (or to taste)

Make the vegetables. While the rice cooks, broth sauté the following ingredients in a large skillet on medium-low heat until the onions are transparent and most of the liquid released by the mushrooms has evaporated, about 8 to 10 minutes.

- 1 medium red, yellow, or white onion, diced (about 1½ cups)
- 2 cloves garlic, finely chopped
- 8 ounces cremini or white button mushrooms, sliced or chopped

Add the following ingredients to the skillet, turn off the heat, and stir gently.

- ⅓ cup roasted pine nuts or pecans
- 1 tablespoon white miso
- ½ teaspoon dried rosemary or 1½ teaspoons fresh rosemary, chopped
- ½ teaspoon dried thyme
- ½ teaspoon dried basil
- ½ teaspoon ground fennel seed

Finish the pilaf. Transfer the skillet mixture into the cooked rice when the rice is done. Stir gently. Taste and add salt and pepper as desired.

(Continued on page 155)

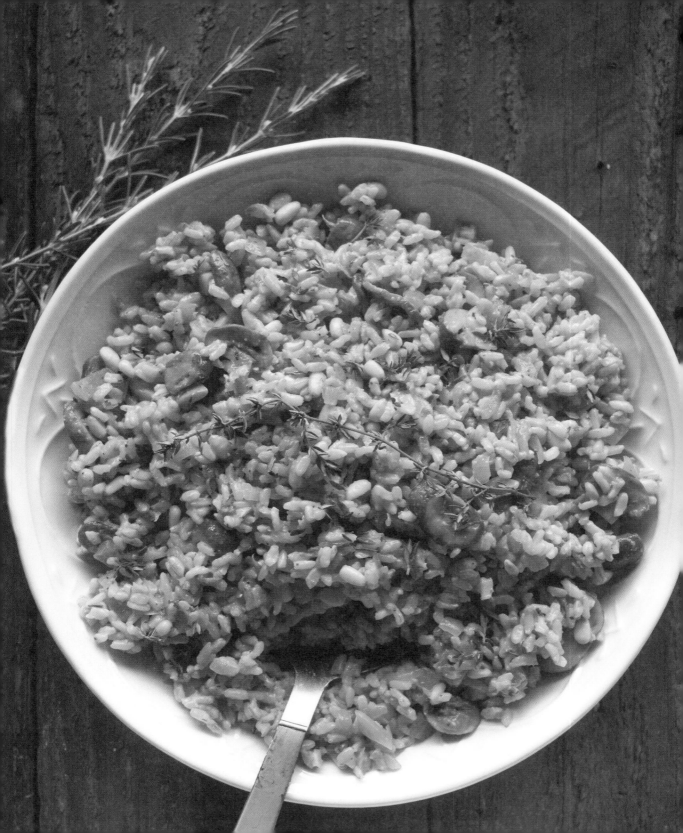

Stovetop directions. Combine the uncooked rice with 3 cups broth and salt (optional) in a medium-large saucepan. Bring to a boil. Cover, reduce the heat to low, and simmer for 45 minutes. Remove the saucepan from the heat and let it sit, covered, for 10 more minutes. While the rice is cooking, make the vegetables as directed above. When the rice is done, fluff it, then transfer the skillet mixture into the cooked rice (or vice versa, whichever pot is bigger) and stir gently. Taste and add salt and pepper as desired.

You can serve the rice with a spoon or shape it into round cakes using an English muffin ring or a large jar lid lined with plastic wrap. This pilaf will keep in the refrigerator for 4 to 5 days. It can be frozen, but I advise using it within a month.

Spanish Brown Rice

Makes 6 servings

This lovely rice gets its color from chili powder, smoked paprika, and ground annatto (also known as achiote), which is available (and inexpensive) at Mexican/Latin grocery stores. The dish is simple to make in an electric pressure cooker, but you can also make it on the stove. It pairs well with Mexican entrees like tacos, tostadas, or Bell Pepper and Mushroom Enchiladas (page 205). Leftover Spanish rice is perfect for burritos, quesadillas, or bowls.

Pressure cooker directions. Add all the ingredients to an electric pressure cooker. Lock the lid. Move the knob to "Sealing." Use the "Multigrain," "Pressure Cook," "High," or "Manual" mode and set for 22 minutes. Wait for 10 minutes after the pressure cooker is done, then move the knob to "Venting" and release the remaining steam before opening the lid.

> **2⅛ cups vegetable broth**
> **1½ cups uncooked brown rice, rinsed**
> **½ cup red, yellow, or white onion, finely chopped**
> **3 cloves garlic, finely chopped**
> **1 teaspoon cumin**
> **1 teaspoon annatto (also known as achiote)**
> **1 teaspoon oregano**
> **¾ teaspoon chili powder**
> **¾ teaspoon smoked paprika**
> **½ teaspoon salt (or to taste)**
> **Freshly ground black pepper to taste**

Stovetop directions. Increase the amount of broth to 3¾ cups. Bring the broth to a boil in a large saucepan or small Dutch oven, then gently stir in all the ingredients. Bring the mixture back to a boil, then reduce the heat to low, cover the pot, and simmer until the rice is tender, 40 to 50 minutes. Remove the pot from the stove and fluff the rice with a fork.

The rice is ready to serve, but it's even better when made ahead of time and cooled, then reheated—the rice is less sticky this way. The rice will keep in the refrigerator for about a week and can be frozen for a month.

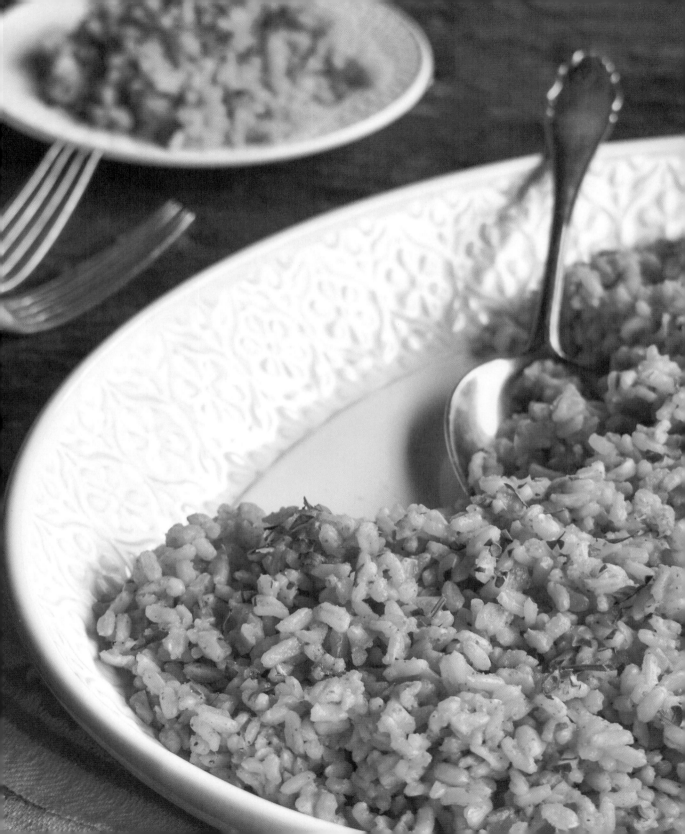

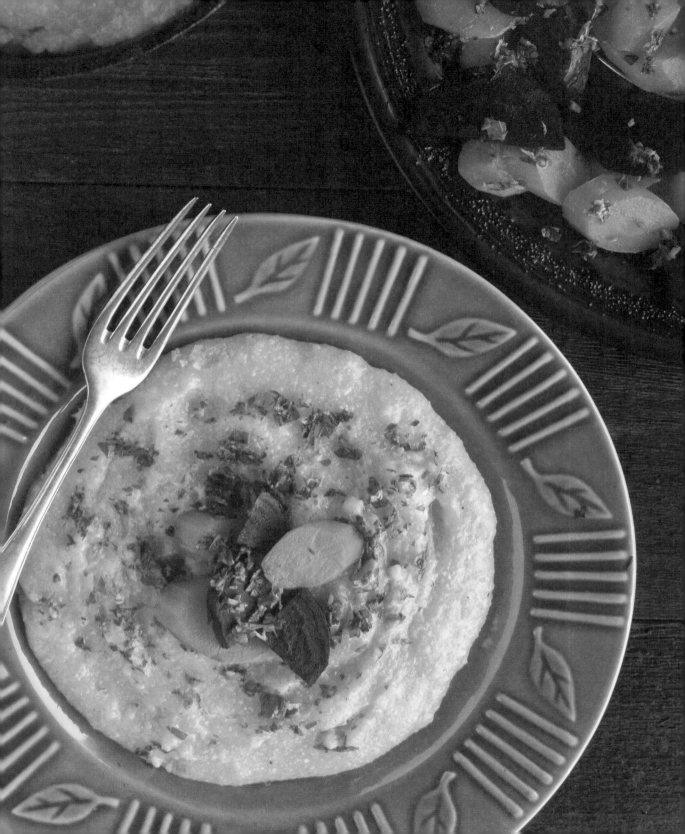

Garlicky Polenta with Gremolata

Makes 8 servings

How a cup of polenta absorbs more than four times its volume in water is a mystery to me, but the result is a moist, fluffy, comforting dish of corn mush. You can serve the polenta right away, similar to mashed potatoes, or you can mold it and eat it later in hardened shapes. It's critically important to whisk the polenta often to avoid lumps. Polenta tastes great drenched in marinara sauce, or sprinkled with gremolata, a traditional parsley-based condiment from Italy. Its bright flavors liven up dishes like cooked grains, pastas, soups, roasted vegetables, and bowls.

Pressure cooker directions. Use a whisk to thoroughly whisk the following ingredients together in an electric pressure cooker.

4½ cups water
1 cup uncooked polenta (not instant)
1 teaspoon salt (or to taste)

Lock the lid. Move the knob to "Sealing." Use the "Pressure Cook," "High," or "Manual" mode and set for 9 minutes. Wait for 10 minutes after the pressure cooker is done, then move the knob to "Venting" and release the remaining steam before opening the lid. Immediately use your whisk to thoroughly delump the polenta, then whisk the following ingredients into the polenta, making sure the entire mixture is homogeneous and creamy.

¼ cup nutritional yeast
½ teaspoon garlic powder
Several grinds of pepper

Stovetop directions. Decrease the water to 4 cups. Bring the water to a boil, add the salt, then, while whisking gently, pour the polenta into the boiling water in a steady stream. Turn down the heat to low and continue whisking until the polenta doesn't drop to the bottom but is thickened and incorporated with the water, a minute or 2. Cover the polenta and continue cooking on low. Stir well every 10 minutes, making sure to get at the sides, bottom, and corners of the pan. Add water if you need to. Cook 30 to 40 minutes—check after 30 minutes to see if you like the texture or if you want a thicker texture, which will take 5 to 10 minutes more. At the end, stir in the nutritional yeast, garlic powder, and pepper.

The polenta is ready to serve and will be similar to stiff mashed potatoes if eaten immediately. It can be served with a sauce or a little gremolata on top (see recipe on next page). Alternatively, spread the polenta into a glass or metal baking dish and refrigerate it. It will gel and can be sliced and served with a sauce. Polenta will keep in the refrigerator for about a week and can be frozen.

Gremolata

Makes about ¼ cup

Wash and dry the parsley. Remove the stems and discard them. Finely chop the leaves until you have about 2–3 tablespoons of chopped parsley.

1 small bunch Italian flat-leaf parsley

In a small bowl, stir together the following ingredients, taste, and season with salt and pepper.

The chopped parsley
1 clove garlic, finely chopped
Zest from 1 lemon
⅛ teaspoon salt (or to taste)
Freshly ground black pepper to taste

The gremolata is ready to serve.

You can also make the gremolata in a food processor. You do not need to chop the parsley leaves. Just add them with the remaining ingredients and pulse in a food processor until everything is finely chopped and well incorporated and seasoned.

The gremolata lasts 4 to 5 days in the refrigerator. It does not freeze well.

Polenta vs. grits vs. cornmeal

All three of these whole grains are made from dried, ground corn, but the differences can be important.

- Polenta is usually made from yellow flint corn, which has a firmer texture than dent corn. Polenta can be milled to a fine or medium texture. Many people put cooked polenta into pans and let it set. It can be served in slices or wedges once it's gelled.
- Grits are mostly available in medium and coarse grinds, usually from white dent corn, which creates a softer texture compared to polenta. Grits are often eaten fresh from the stove when they are soft and creamy.
- Cornmeal comes from white or yellow corn and is usually bought in a fine grind (although it comes in various textures). Cornmeal can be cooked into "mush" but it's more often used in baked goods.

Curried Amaranth Patties

Makes 9 large or 18 small cakes

The tiny grain amaranth comes out thick and a bit gooey for my taste when prepared as a hot cereal for breakfast. I prefer it in these patties, where it's combined with greens, beans, oats, vegetables, and Indian spices. I love the firm texture that comes from baking the patties—no mushy burgers here. You could serve these patties with rice and a curry sauce or chutney. They could also be served crumbled in an Indian-inspired bowl or on a bun, hamburger-style, with Indian-inspired toppings, including chutney stirred into plant-based mayonnaise.

Preheat the oven to 425°F. Line a sheet pan with parchment paper or a silicone mat.

Cook the amaranth. In a medium saucepan, stir together the following ingredients and bring to a boil. Then, reduce the heat to low, cover, and simmer until the amaranth is tender and very thick (thicker than oatmeal), 15 to 20 minutes. Remove from the heat and set aside.

> **1 cup water**
> **½ cup uncooked amaranth**

Prep the chia seeds. In a small bowl, fork-whisk the following ingredients together. The mixture will be very thick. Set aside.

> **¼ cup water**
> **1 tablespoon chia seeds, ground in a small blender, coffee grinder, or spice grinder**

Water sauté the vegetables. While the amaranth is cooking, water sauté the following ingredients in a medium skillet until the onion is soft and transparent, 8 to 10 minutes.

> **1 small red, yellow, or white onion, diced (about 1 cup)**
> **4 cloves garlic, chopped**

Once the onion is tender, add the spinach or chard to the skillet and stir until wilted, 1 to 2 minutes. Turn off the heat and set aside.

> **1 cup spinach or Swiss chard, chopped**

Combine everything and bake. Put the beans in a large mixing bowl and mash them a bit with a potato masher or pastry cutter.

> **1 (15-ounce) can small red, kidney, or black beans, drained and rinsed**

(Continued on page 163)

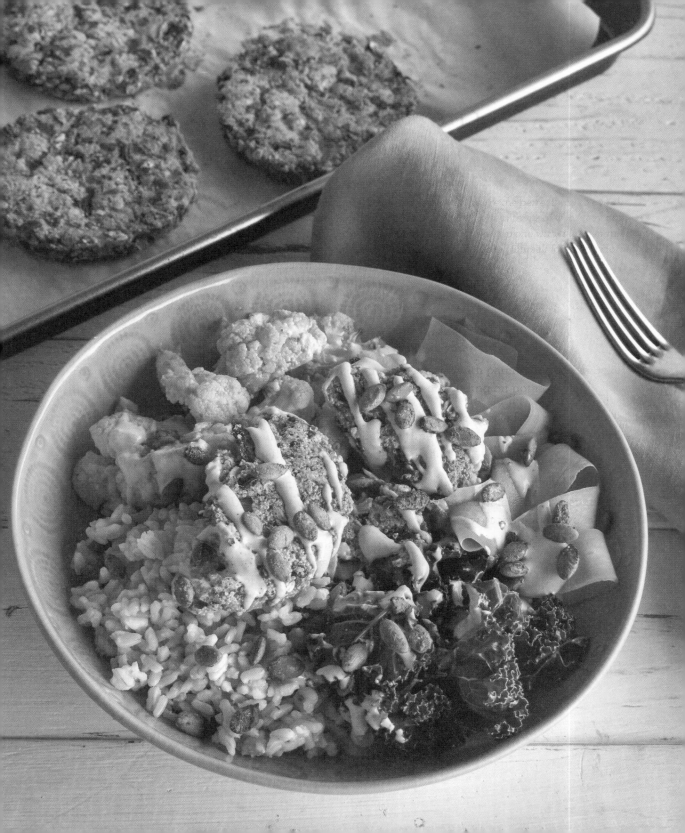

Add the following ingredients to the bowl and combine them with the beans.

The cooked amaranth
The chia seed mixture
The skillet mixture
⅓ cup quick cooking oats or dried whole grain breadcrumbs
⅓ cup fresh cilantro, chopped
1 tablespoon chili powder or 1 or more teaspoons Kashmiri chili powder
2 teaspoons coriander
1½ teaspoons fresh ginger, finely chopped
1 teaspoon cumin
1 teaspoon turmeric
1 teaspoon garam masala
¼ teaspoon salt (or to taste)
Pinch red pepper flakes (or to taste)

For large patties, form 3- to 4-inch disks (fairly thin) with your hands; for small patties, make them 2 inches wide. (The mixture will be sticky. Wet your hands if needed.) Lay the patties on your lined pan. Bake for 20 minutes, then flip them over and bake 15 minutes more or until firm and dark golden brown.

The amaranth patties are ready to serve. They will last in the refrigerator for about a week. They freeze well.

Savory Quinoa Cakes

Makes 7 servings

For many years these cakes have served as my plant-based centerpiece for Thanksgiving. They pair incredibly well with mushroom gravy or easy vegan gravy (see graciousvegan.com for gravy recipes), and produce a distinct autumn vibe with their parsley, thyme, and mushroom flavors. When not serving a crowd, I like to freeze the leftovers and take out a few cakes every now and then for lunch or dinner. They go well with side vegetables and any of the grain dishes in this cookbook.

Preheat the oven to 350°F and line a sheet pan with parchment paper (do not use a silicone mat, because the cakes tend to stick to the mat).

Toast the walnuts. Spread the walnuts on the sheet pan and bake them until they just start to change color and you can smell the aroma. Start checking after 5 minutes to see if they're done. Remove and cool, then finely chop them in a food processor by pulsing multiple times—do not let them turn into walnut butter. Set aside and turn off the oven.

½ cup walnuts

Cook the potato. Prick the potato in several places with a fork, then microwave it until soft, 3 to 5 minutes. Rinse under cold water so it is cool enough to handle, then cut it open, scoop out the flesh, and roughly mash it in a large bowl.

1 medium russet, red, or Yukon gold potato

Sauté the onions and mushrooms. In a large skillet, Dutch oven, or other large pan, water sauté the onions and mushrooms until the onion is tender and transparent and the water released by the mushrooms has evaporated, 8 to 10 minutes.

1 small red, yellow, or white onion, diced (about 1 cup)
4 medium or large white button or cremini mushrooms, finely chopped (this can be done in the food processor)

Put it all together and broil. Add the following ingredients to the potato mixture in the large bowl and stir everything until combined. Do not mash or puree.

The toasted walnuts
The onions and mushrooms
2 cups cooked quinoa (use the Whole Grains Cooking Guide on page 43)

(Continued on page 166)

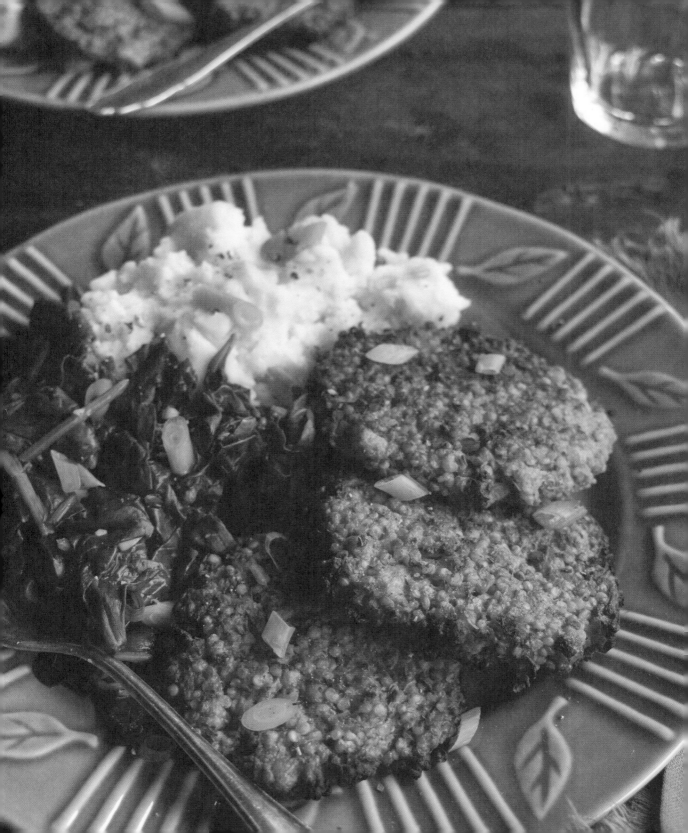

⅓ cup flour of choice

¼ cup fresh parsley, finely chopped

1 teaspoon thyme

¾ teaspoon salt (or to taste)

½ teaspoon paprika

Right before cooking, stir the whipped tofu into the quinoa mixture.

¾ cup silken tofu, whipped until smooth in a food processor

Shape the mixture into 12 to 16 cakes and lay them on the sheet pan. Position an oven rack about 5 inches from the broiler and turn the broiler to high (500°F). Broil the cakes for 4 minutes, until golden brown on top. Flip them over and broil 2 minutes more or until golden brown.

The quinoa cakes are ready to serve. They will last about a week in the refrigerator, and they freeze well.

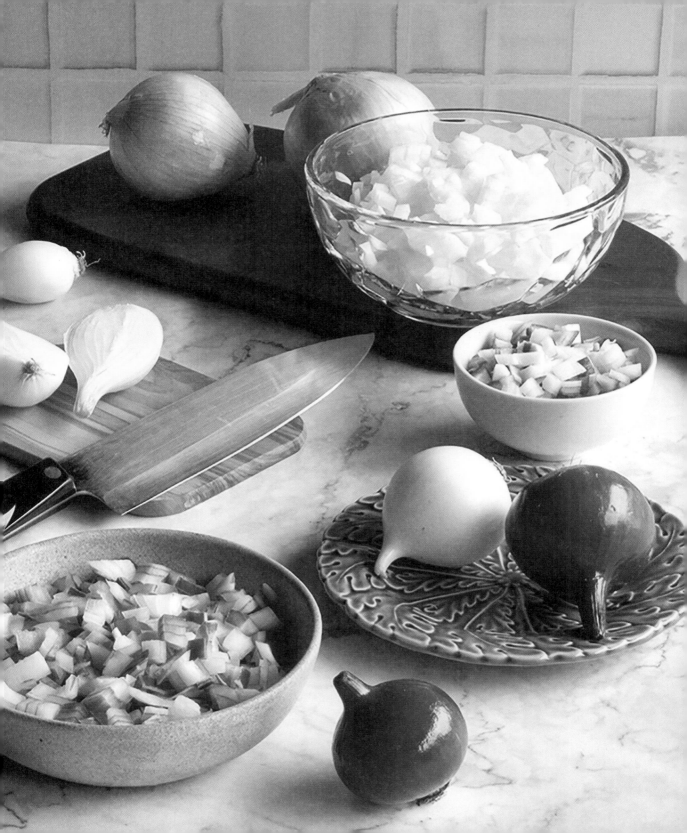

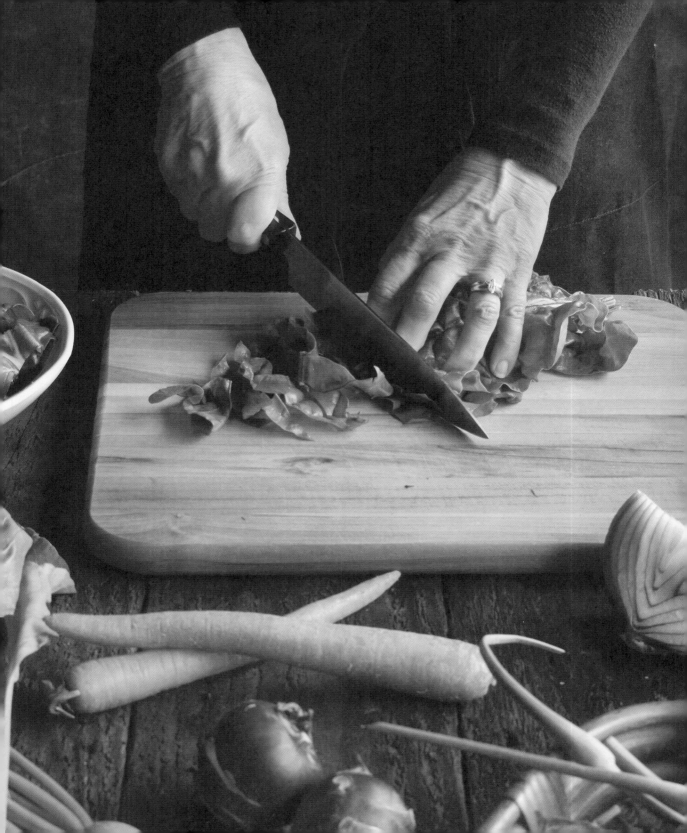

Vegetables

For plant-based eaters, the line between side dish and entree can be blurry. One person's side dish, like Eggplant Parmesan Stacks (page 190), is another person's entree when served with a side of Italian Chopped Salad with Sun-Dried Tomato Dressing (page 94). Labels like side dish or entree don't matter. It's all good.

In this chapter, I include dishes centered around a particular star vegetable like eggplant or red cabbage, or on a preparation technique like roasting, pickling, pureeing, or stir-frying without oil. You be the judge as to whether to serve them as an entree, side dish, lunch, or dinner (with leftovers for breakfast always being a possibility).

If you get a farm share or have your own vegetable garden, some of these recipes, like Creamy Pureed Greens (page 178), may come in quite handy.

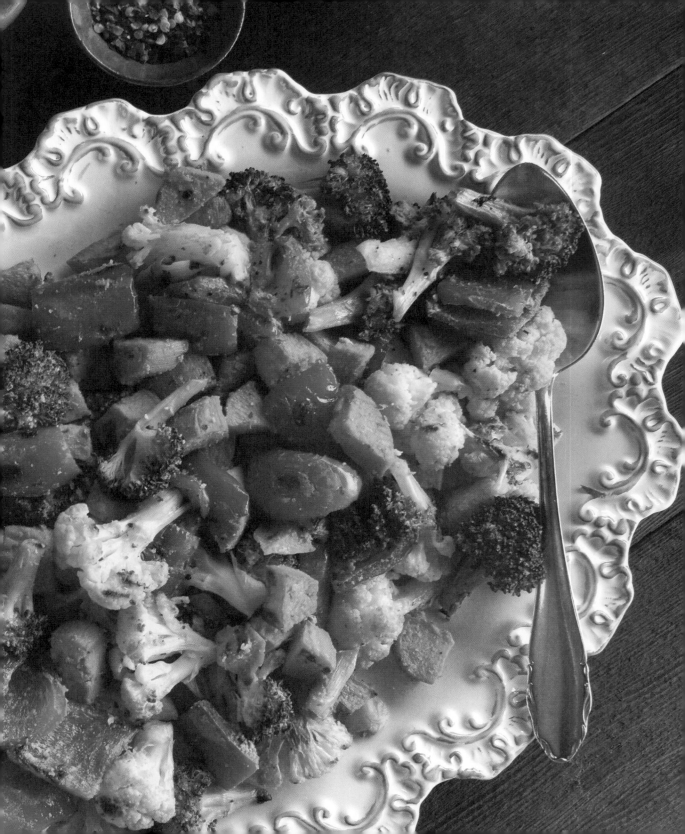

Roasting Vegetables without Oil

Makes 4 servings

Many of my students like to roast up a few batches of vegetables on the weekend so that they can grab them on busy weeknights when cooking from scratch just isn't possible. But all that oil can add empty calories so I found an easy way to make roasted vegetables using tahini, water, and savory spices. High oven heat and parchment paper are essential. If you want to use another spice combination, eliminate the onion powder, garlic powder, and smoked paprika, and substitute a teaspoon of your preferred spices.

Preheat the oven to 425°F or 450°F (if your oven runs hot, I recommend 425°F). Line a sheet pan with parchment paper (or just go with an unlined pan). Whisk the following ingredients together in a large bowl.

5 teaspoons water
4 teaspoons tahini
½ teaspoon salt (or to taste)
⅛ teaspoon onion powder
⅛ teaspoon garlic powder
Pinch smoked paprika

Add in the following ingredients and fold with a spatula until all the cubes are coated.

1 pound vegetables, cut into chunks, cubes, florets, or slices (note that for potatoes, the tahini mixture covers 1½ pounds)

Transfer the coated vegetables to the lined pan. Roast for half the time (see chart below), then stir the vegetables, rotate the pan, and roast for the remaining time or longer until desired tenderness is reached. The roasted vegetables are ready to eat. They will last 4 to 5 days in the refrigerator but will not be as crispy. They don't freeze well.

Roasting Times

- Root vegetables (potatoes, turnips, beets, parsnips, carrots): 24 to 40 minutes
- Winter squash (butternut, acorn, delicata, etc.): 25 to 40 minutes
- Cruciferous (**cauliflower, broccoli, Brussels sprouts, cabbage, kale**): 15 to 25 minutes
- Watery vegetables (**eggplant**, **red bell peppers**, other bell peppers, zucchini and other summer squash, **red onions**, **garlic**, green beans, asparagus): 10 to 20 minutes

(Continued on page 172)

Spice combinations for roasted vegetables

- Old Bay seasoning
- Montreal steak seasoning or other favorite seasoning mix
- Spike seasoning
- Cajun seasoning
- Smoked paprika
- Fresh thyme and **rosemary**, chopped (optional to add fresh **garlic**, finely chopped)
- Balsamic vinegar
- Sesame oil, **garlic powder**, red pepper flakes
- **Curry powder**

Baked Spring Rolls

Makes 16 (4-inch) rolls

I've yet to find spring roll or wonton wrappers made of whole grain flour so I use whole wheat flour tortillas and bake or air fry these baked spring rolls for a crispy, healthy appetizer or side dish. This recipe is easy to scale up or down. The maple syrup-based dipping sauce adds even more nuance to the flavor combination. You can choose your favorite vegetables for the filling, although I recommend always including garlic, onions, and mushrooms.

Baking directions. Preheat the oven to 425°F. Line a sheet pan with parchment paper or a silicone mat.

Water sauté the following ingredients in a wok, large skillet, or other large pan until the vegetables are just tender and the pan is dry, 8 to 12 minutes.

> **6 cups shredded or finely chopped vegetables such as red bell peppers, other bell peppers, bok choy, broccoli, cabbage, carrots, celery, garlic, mushrooms, green onions, red onion, green onions, and water chestnuts**
> **2 tablespoons fresh cilantro, chopped**
> **4 teaspoons fresh ginger, finely chopped**

Add the following ingredients and cook for 1 to 2 minutes, until the mixture is nicely mixed and mostly dry.

> **3 tablespoons soy sauce or tamari**
> **1 tablespoon maple syrup**
> **4 teaspoons Chinese roasted sesame paste (see box page 131) or sesame oil**
> **1 teaspoon rice vinegar or other white vinegar**
> **½–1 teaspoon chili-garlic paste, sriracha, or other chili sauce**

To create the rolls, put ⅛ of the mixture on a tortilla, then roll it up tightly and place it seam side down on the sheet pan. Repeat with the remaining tortillas.

> **8 (8-inch) whole wheat flour tortillas**

Bake until golden, 13 to 15 minutes. Cut each roll in half and serve with the Maple Sesame Dipping Sauce (recipe on page 175) or your favorite sauce.

(Continued on page 175)

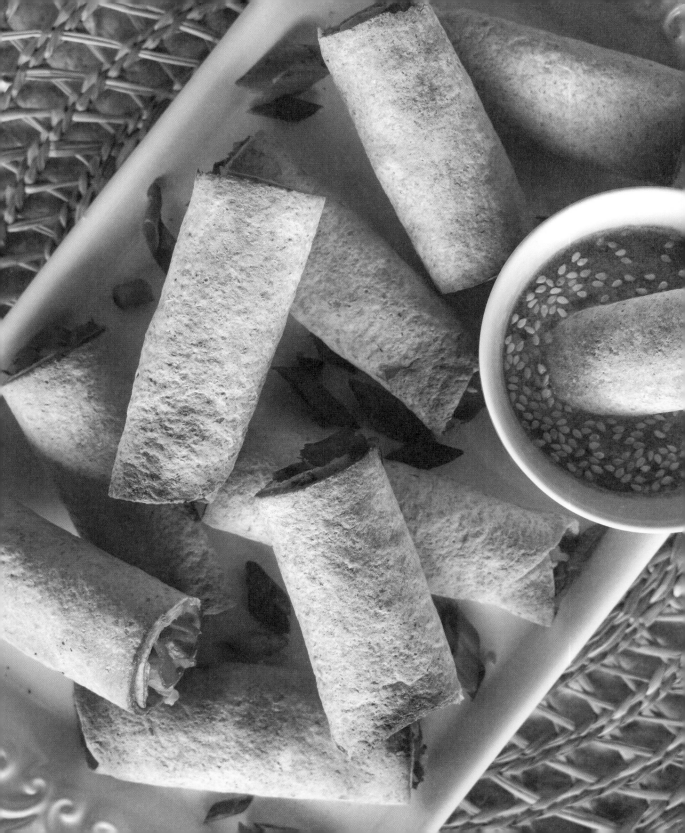

Air frying directions. Rather than baking the rolls in the oven, lay them in an air fryer in a single layer and air fry at 400°F for 7 minutes, turning the rolls over halfway through. Add more minutes until they are golden. (I cut them in half before air frying them because my air fryer is small.)

The rolls will last in the refrigerator for about a week. They will crisp up best if you bake or air fry them after they've been refrigerated. They can be frozen.

Maple Sesame Dipping Sauce

Add the following ingredients to a jar, put on the lid, and shake them together.

¼ cup maple syrup
2 tablespoons soy sauce or tamari
1 teaspoon Chinese roasted sesame paste (see box on page 131) or sesame oil
1 teaspoon rice wine vinegar
½ teaspoon fresh ginger, finely chopped

The dipping sauce is ready to use. It can be stored in the refrigerator for up to a week.

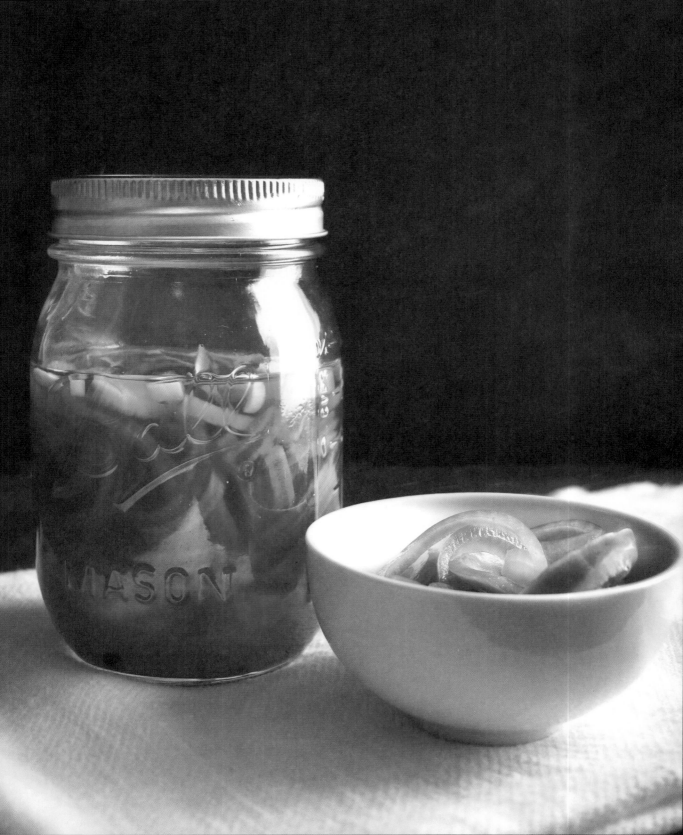

Pickled Red Onions

Makes about 2 cups pickled onions

These neon-pink rings look "wow!" and taste even better. The vinegar mixture saps the raw onions of their pungent sting, letting the delicious sour taste of the onion come through. Pickled onion rings are great on hummus or avocado toast, scrambled tofu, tacos, tostadas, burritos, all kinds of sandwiches, and many salads. They add color, crispness, and their own special zing to bowls, too.

Peel the onion, thinly slice it into ⅛-inch rings, and place them in a 2-cup pint jar with a lid. Set aside.

1 medium red onion

In a small saucepan, stir together the following ingredients. Bring to a boil and stir until the salt dissolves.

¾ cup water
½ cup white distilled vinegar or ¼ cup white distilled vinegar and ¼ cup apple cider vinegar
4 whole peppercorns
3 dried bay leaves
2 tablespoons maple syrup
1¼ teaspoons salt (or to taste)

Turn off the heat. Allow the mixture to cool for about 5 minutes, then pour the liquid over the onions in the jar. With a spoon, press down on the onions to make sure they are submerged.

Close the lid on the jar (leaving it slightly ajar), let it cool to room temperature, then put the jar in the refrigerator. The pickled onions are best starting the next day, but even after a few hours they are good. They last about 1 month in the fridge. They do not freeze well.

Creamy Pureed Greens

Makes about 2½ cups puree

This is a puree that can be used on baked potatoes, crackers, bread, pasta, or pizza; as part of a bowl or quesadilla; or snuggled next to stewed tomatoes, mashed potatoes, or rice pilaf as a side dish. I used to make this dish with collard greens only, but I've found more recently that it works with any combination of dark, leafy greens. You can make a smaller batch of this recipe, but my large blender only works well with the amounts listed here (or doubled). A food processor can handle smaller batches, but the result will likely not be as smooth as with a blender.

Trim and steam the greens. If the leaves are large, cut them in half or quarters. (You can either compost the stems or finely slice them and add them to the mix.)

> **About 1½ pounds dark, leafy greens (collard, mustard, turnip, radish, beetchard, bok choy, kale, spinach)**

Steam the greens. I use my pressure cooker (see "Steaming Vegetables in the Instant Pot" on graciousvegan.com for more information) but you can also steam or boil the greens on the stove (cooking times range from 1 minute for spinach, 2 minutes for chard, to 10 minutes for collards and kale; check that the greens are tender but have not lost their bright green color).

Make the puree. Transfer the drained, steamed greens to a blender or food processor. Add the following ingredients to the greens.

> **1 tablespoon tahini**
> **1 tablespoon nutritional yeast**
> **1 teaspoon garlic powder**
> **1 teaspoon salt (or to taste)**

Process the mixture until a puree texture is reached. You may need to add a little water, and you may need to stop and scrape down the sides once or twice. The greens are ready to serve. They will keep in the refrigerator for 4 to 5 days. They freeze well.

The Plant-Based Anti-Inflammatory Cookbook

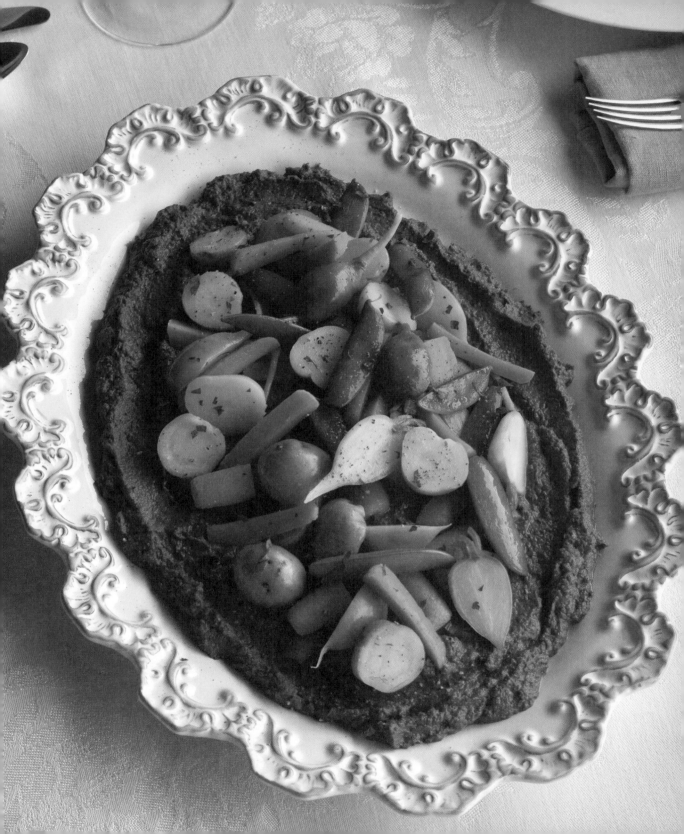

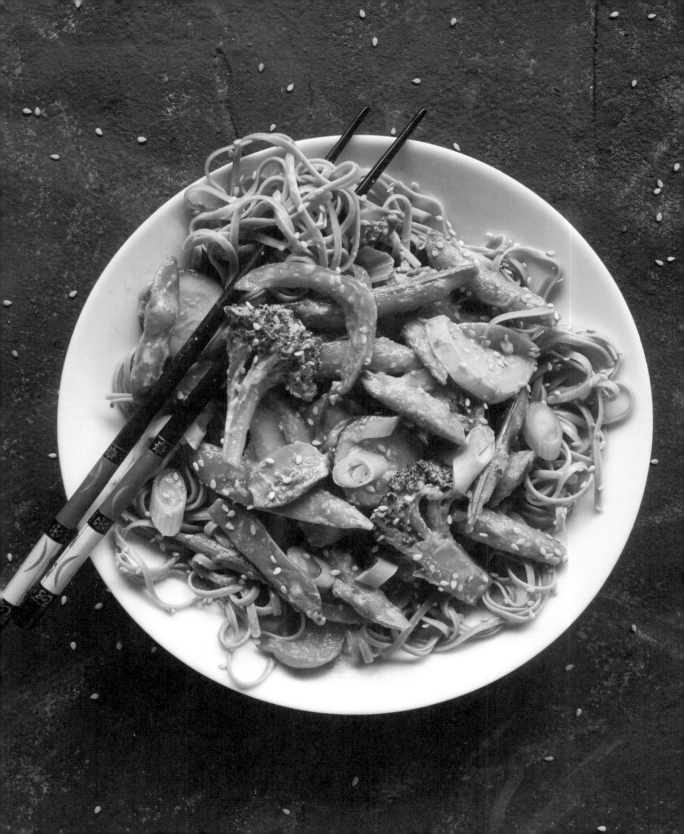

Stir-Fried Sugar Snap Peas

🌱

Makes 4 servings

I used to enjoy sugar snap peas exclusively as a raw snack with other vegetable sticks. But what a pleasant surprise when I started cooking them! Sugar snap peas star in this stir-fry, but they can be included in any stir-fry, either whole or sliced. This versatile stir-fry sauce brings ginger, garlic, miso, sesame, and chili flavors to the party, and you can control the spice levels. Sometimes I serve this stir-fry with rice, and sometimes I add in cooked soba noodles right at the end and have a noodle stir-fry.

Make the stir-fry sauce. Whisk the following ingredients together in a jar or bowl or use a small blender to get everything well incorporated. Set aside.

- **2 tablespoons white miso**
- **2 tablespoons soy sauce or tamari**
- **2 tablespoons water**
- **1 tablespoon fresh ginger, finely chopped**
- **1 tablespoon maple syrup or 2 Medjool dates**
- **1 tablespoon Chinese roasted sesame paste (see box on page 131) or sesame oil**
- **2 cloves garlic, finely chopped**
- **Pinch crushed red pepper flakes**

Make the stir-fry. Use a wok, very large nonstick skillet, or Dutch oven. Water sauté the following ingredients until they are cooked to your desired firmness and any sauté water is evaporated, 4 to 8 minutes.

- **8 ounces (about 3 cups) whole sugar snap peas**
- **5 cups vegetables such as chopped asparagus, broccoli, yellow or green zucchini, mushrooms, bean sprouts, water chestnuts, and green cabbage or thinly sliced carrots, red bell peppers, and other bell peppers**

After the vegetables are tender-firm to your liking, stir in the sauce and cook for 2 to 4 minutes, until the sauce is bubbling and all the vegetables are coated.

Serve on rice or noodles.

- **Cooked brown rice or cooked noodles (e.g., buckwheat soba noodles)**

Garnish with green onions and sesame seeds, if desired.

- **3–4 green onions, sliced on the diagonal**
- **1 tablespoon roasted sesame seeds**

This stir-fry will last 4 to 5 days in the refrigerator (store the vegetables separately from the rice). This dish does not freeze well.

Red Cabbage with Walnuts and Olives

Makes 6 servings

Cabbage, onions, apple, olives, and walnuts together? Yes, it works! My students have been pleasantly surprised by this recipe. The sweet and sour flavors from apple, cabbage, and onions are mellowed by cooking them down, then olives and vinegar bring last-minute sharpness and brininess. With six anti-inflammatory superstars, this dish is a winner from a health perspective. It thrives in combination with a cooked grain or potato or you could serve it with a mellow entree like Stuffed Bell Pepper Rings (page 199), Asparagus with Orzo and Breadcrumbs (page 216), or a creamy pasta.

Toast the walnuts. Turn on the oven to 350°F. (You don't have to wait until it's preheated.) Spread the walnuts in a single layer on a baking sheet or pan. Bake 8 to 10 minutes (fewer minutes if the oven is preheated) until the pieces are light golden brown and aromatic. Set aside and turn off the oven.

⅓ cup walnuts, roughly chopped

Make the dish. Add the following ingredients to a Dutch oven or other large pan. Cook the vegetables on medium-low, covered, for 5 minutes, then remove the cover and cook about 5 minutes more, until the water is evaporated and the ingredients are just tender.

1 pound (5–6 cups) **red cabbage**, thinly sliced or shredded
1 **red apple** (unpeeled), cored and thinly sliced
½ large **red onion**, thinly sliced
1 clove **garlic**, finely chopped
¼ cup water

Add the following ingredients and stir just enough to combine. Remove from heat.

The toasted walnuts
⅓ cup Greek or Kalamata **olives**, sliced
1 tablespoon sherry vinegar, white wine vinegar, or champagne vinegar (see box on page 88)
1 tablespoon fresh **parsley**, chopped, or 1 teaspoon dried
1 tablespoon fresh marjoram, chopped, or 1 teaspoon dried
½ teaspoon salt (or to taste)
Freshly ground black pepper to taste

The dish is ready to serve. It will keep in the refrigerator for 4 to 5 days. It does not freeze well.

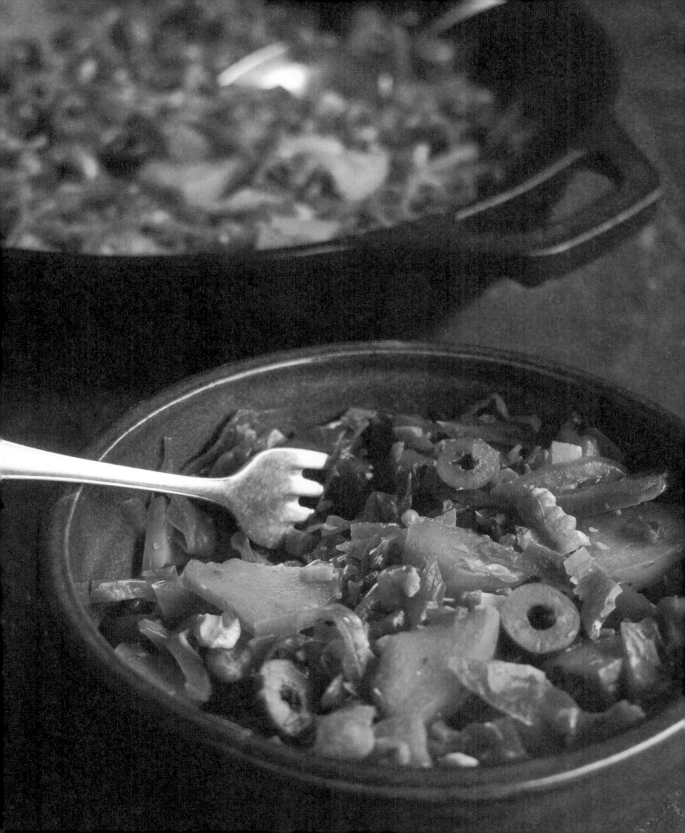

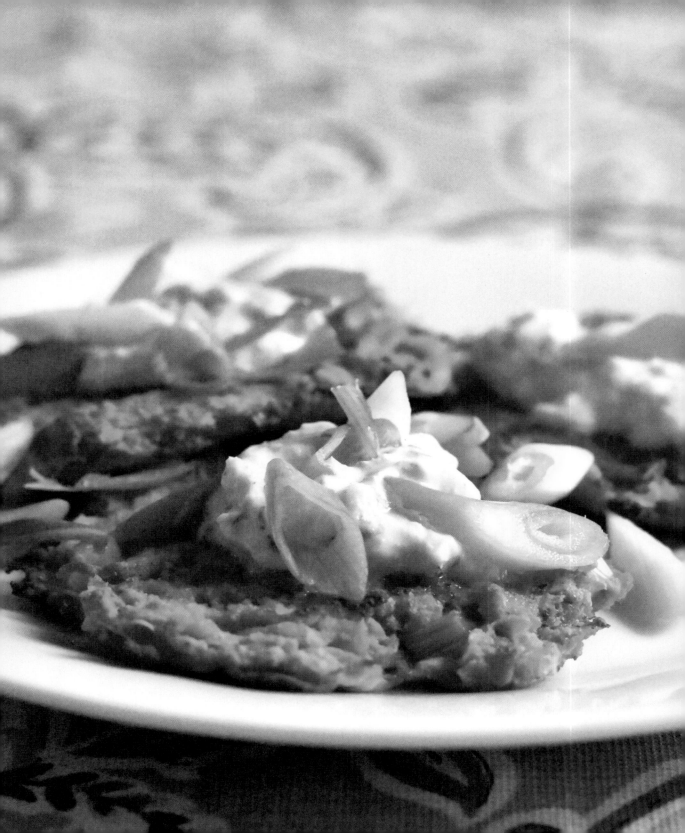

Sweet Potato Cakes

Makes 16 cakes (5 servings)

This recipe looks a little fussy at first glance, calling for both baked and grated raw sweet potatoes, but it results in beautiful, tasty sweet potato cakes with a light texture. Once you make it a few times, it becomes routine. The cakes make a great side dish for a special dinner or they can take center stage with a cooked grain and topping like plant-based tzatziki, sour cream, or any sauce you like. Sweet potato cakes could also go in a sandwich or burrito.

Preheat the oven to 425°F. Line two large sheet pans with parchment paper (do not use silicone mats because the cakes stick to them).

Prep the potatoes. Poke 1 sweet potato with the point of a knife in a few places to allow air to escape, then microwave on high for 3 to 5 minutes or until soft. Scoop out the flesh into a bowl and mash it. Grate the other 2 raw sweet potatoes. Set aside.

3 sweet potatoes (1½ pounds), divided

Prep the "egg." Blend the following ingredients together in a small blender or with a stick (immersion) blender. Set aside

⅓ cup unsweetened nondairy milk
¼ cup water
1 tablespoon cornstarch or 2 tablespoons whole wheat flour
⅛ teaspoon baking powder
⅛ teaspoon turmeric

Make the mixture and bake. In a large bowl, stir together the following ingredients until well combined.

The mashed and grated sweet potatoes
The "egg"
4 green onions, thinly sliced
½ cup dried whole grain breadcrumbs
¾ teaspoon salt (or to taste)
½ teaspoon baking powder
¼ teaspoon garlic powder

Create potato cakes by laying rounded 2-tablespoon scoops of the mixture on the sheet pan and flattening them with your hand. Bake 20 minutes, then flip them over. Bake another 10 minutes or until golden. The sweet potato cakes are ready to serve. They keep in the refrigerator for about a week. They can be frozen. I recommend topping with plant-based sour cream (see graciousvegan.com for a recipe).

Baked Sweet Potatoes with Easy, Tasty Toppings

Makes as many servings as you like

Baked sweet potatoes can form the basis of countless quick lunches or dinners. They're the perfect way to avoid having to order takeout. I provide some ideas for toppings below, but the sky's the limit in terms of what they pair well with. Find your favorites. Baked sweet potatoes make an excellent breakfast, too—top one with a little maple syrup, cinnamon, flaxseed meal, and nuts and you've found a quick and easy way to fuel yourself for a long morning. Add some cooked grains or plant-based yogurt if you like.

Bake the sweet potatoes. Wash, dry, and pierce each sweet potato in several places with a fork or pointed knife.

Purple sweet potatoes or orange sweet potatoes (as many as you want)

For oven baking, place the sweet potatoes on a baking sheet lined with parchment paper. Bake until tender at 425°F for 40 to 50 minutes. Baking times vary depending on potato size.

For microwave baking, wrap each sweet potato in a paper towel. Microwave for 3 minutes, check it, then cook for a minute at a time until just tender. Baking times will vary depending on your oven, how many potatoes you bake together, and the size of the potatoes.

Top the potatoes. Before cutting open the potato, cradle it in a towel and gently knead it with your hands to soften the insides. Use a knife or fork to make a long slit in the potato, then open the potato for serving. Top with one of the suggested topping combinations below or toppings of your choice.

Black beans and salsa (guacamole optional)
Chili beans and vegan sour cream, crema, or guacamole
Cowboy caviar (a mixture of black-eyed peas, corn, avocado, tomatoes, red onions, cilantro, and a little vinegar and salt)
Chickpeas, chopped tomatoes, and cucumber with tahini sauce
Leftover chili
Cooked vegetables with leftover sauce (peanut sauce, curry sauce, pesto)
Pomegranate molasses, vegan sour cream or crema, and an interesting dried spice like dukkah, za'atar, urfa biber, or Aleppo pepper

Recipes for vegan sour cream, vegan crema, guacamole, chili, tahini sauce, peanut sauce, curry sauce, pesto, gravy, dukkah, and za'atar are available on graciousvegan.com.

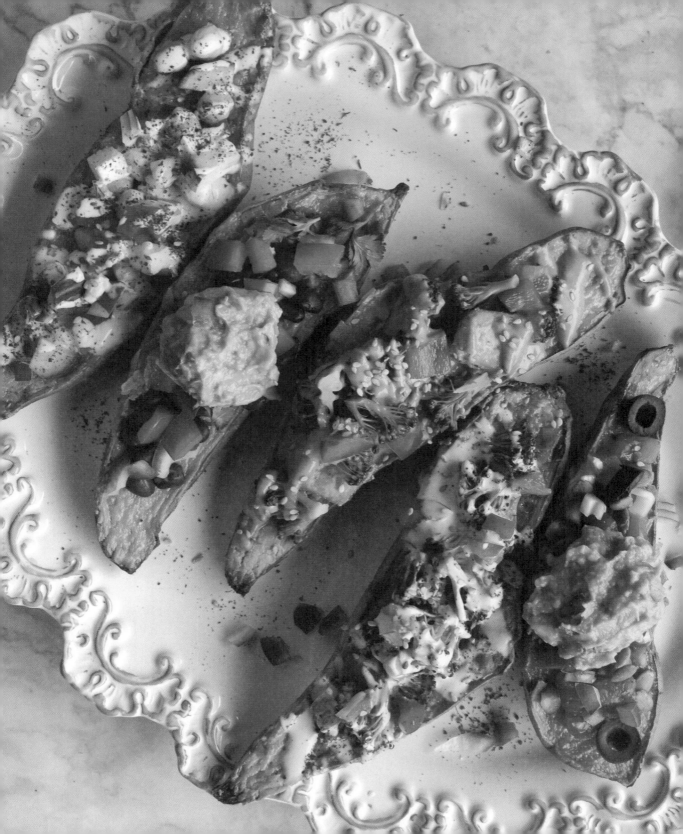

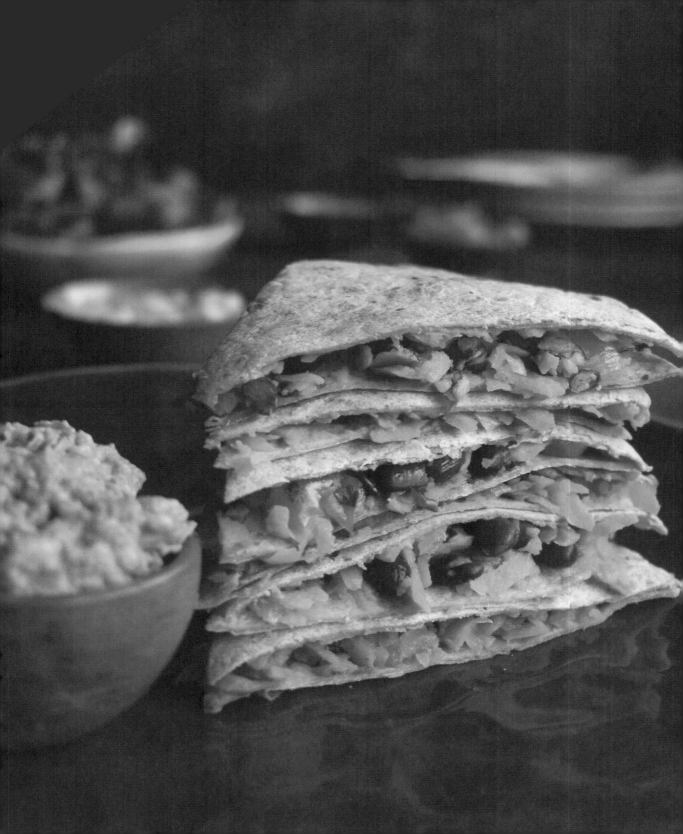

Spicy Sweet Potato Chipotle Quesadillas with Guacamole

Makes 5 servings

So few ingredients, such great taste. The combination here makes for a perfect quesadilla filling in both taste—spicy, but also sweet and savory—and texture—not mushy, but it sticks together well. Top these quesadillas with homemade guacamole, and you've got a party in your mouth!

Water sauté the following ingredients in a large skillet or Dutch oven until the vegetables are just tender, 8 to 10 minutes.

12–13 ounces sweet potato, peeled and grated (about 3 cups)
1 (15-ounce) can black beans, drained and rinsed
½ medium red, yellow, or white onion, diced (about ¾ cup)
½ red bell pepper, diced

Stir in the following ingredients and remove the pan from the heat.

3–4 tablespoons fresh cilantro, chopped
¼–½ teaspoon or more chipotle chili powder or chipotle peppers from 1 can chipotle peppers in adobo sauce, finely diced
½ teaspoon salt (or to taste)

Spread a fifth of the mixture onto half of each tortilla, then fold the tortillas in half. Cook the quesadillas on a griddle or in a dry skillet until light brown on the first side, then flip them and cook them on the second side until light brown.

5 (8-inch) whole wheat flour tortillas

Serve with guacamole. (Guacamole recipe is available on graciousvegan.com.)

The quesadilla filling lasts for about a week in the refrigerator. It can be frozen.

Eggplant Parmesan Stacks

Makes 6 side-dish servings or 3 main-dish servings

August and September bring a bumper crop of eggplants to gardens and farmers' markets, meaning this recipe is a winner in late summer and early fall. I skip breading and frying the eggplants in favor of oil-free roasting. The dark purple eggplant peel contains anti-inflammatory anthocyanins, so leave the peel on if at all possible. You could make this into a casserole rather than stacks if you wish. The stacks work well as a side dish or entree.

Prep the eggplant. Preheat the oven to 475°F (or 450°F if your oven runs hot). Line two sheet pans with parchment paper. Slice the eggplants into ¼- to ½-inch disks (12 or more slices per eggplant).

2 (1-pound) eggplants, unpeeled

Lay the eggplant slices on the pans in a single layer.

Coat the eggplant. In a measuring cup or other small bowl, whisk the following ingredients together.

⅓ **cup water**
¼ **cup tahini**
1 **teaspoon salt (or to taste)**
½ **teaspoon onion powder**
½ **teaspoon garlic powder**
¼ **teaspoon smoked paprika**

Brush both sides of each eggplant slice with the coating. Roast the slices in the oven for 15 minutes. Flip and roast another 12 minutes or until they are golden brown and soft. When they are done, lower the oven temperature to 375°F.

Assemble and bake the stacks. Using an oval or rectangular casserole dish (approximately 11 × 7 inches), spread a thin layer of tomato sauce in the bottom.

2 cups store-bought or homemade marinara sauce (see graciousvegan.com for a recipe)

Lay 6 eggplant disks on the first layer of tomato sauce. Top each with a spoonful of marinara and sprinkling of vegan Parmesan.

½ **cup vegan Parmesan (see graciousvegan.com for a recipe)**

Lay another disk onto each of the 6 disks and top each with marinara and Parmesan. Repeat until all disks are used. Sprinkle any remaining Parmesan on top. Bake uncovered for 25 to 30 minutes, until the sauce is bubbly and the top layer of Parmesan is darker. The stacks are ready to serve. Leftovers will keep in the refrigerator 4 to 5 days. The stacks do not freeze well.

The Plant-Based Anti-Inflammatory Cookbook

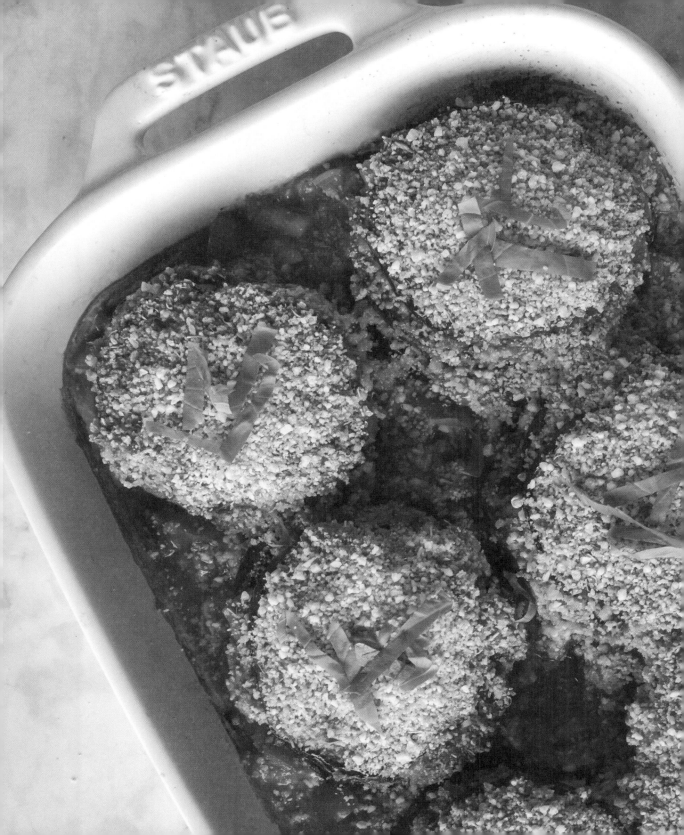

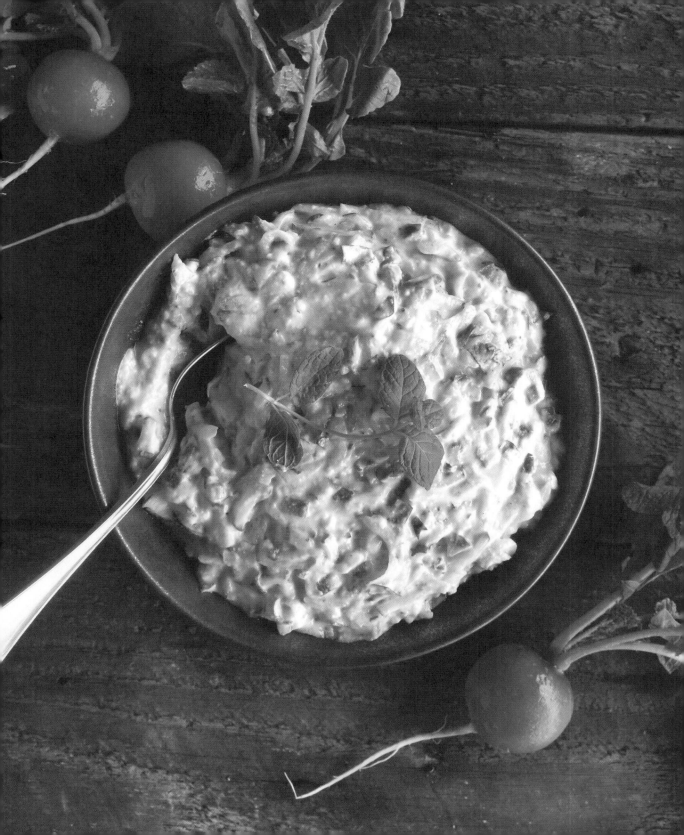

Radish Raita

Makes 2½ cups (6 servings)

Raita is a staple in Indian cuisine because the yogurt in raita helps cool the tongue after eating spicy curries. The humble radish hardly ever serves as the main ingredient in a recipe, so here's my effort to right that wrong. The grated radishes add a crispy texture and a tasty zest, complementing the smooth, cool, plant-based yogurt. This wonderful side dish pairs well with curry and rice or it can be part of an Indian-inspired bowl (do not heat the raita). It also complements the Curried Amaranth Patties on page 161 incredibly well.

Fold together the following ingredients in a medium bowl. Taste, adjust seasonings, and add more yogurt if you like a creamier texture.

- **1½ cups unsweetened vegan yogurt or more if desired***
- **1¼–1½ cups (2 bunches) red or purple radishes, grated****
- **⅓ cup fresh mint and/or cilantro, chopped**
- **½–1 serrano or jalapeño pepper, seeded and deveined (if desired) and finely chopped**
- **3 tablespoons red onion, finely chopped**
- **1 tablespoon fresh lime juice**
- **½ teaspoon cumin**
- **½ teaspoon coriander**
- **⅛ teaspoon salt (or to taste)**

The raita is ready to serve. It will last 24 to 48 hours in the refrigerator. It does not freeze well.

---

* If using homemade yogurt, I recommend straining it beforehand, otherwise water will separate as the raita sits.
** The radishes will release water if you do not eat the raita right after making it. You can always drain off the water if you eat it later, or you can extract water from the grated radishes before you make the raita by grating the radishes, putting the shreds in a colander, sprinkling with about ½ teaspoon salt, stirring it in, and letting the grated radishes sit for about 30 minutes. Then, rinse the radish shreds, put them between several layers of paper towels or a clean kitchen towel, dry them as much as possible, and proceed with the recipe, omitting the salt.

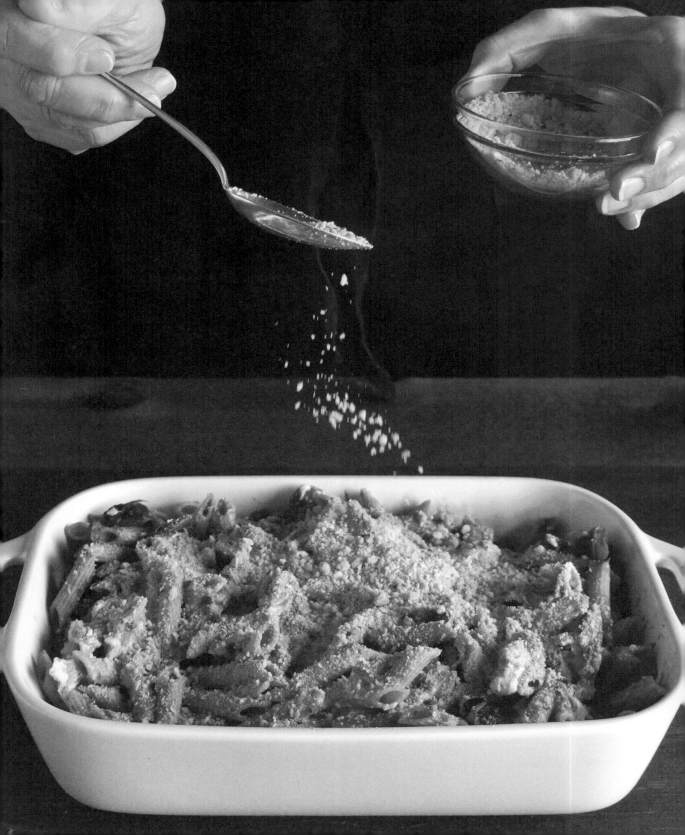

Main Dishes

The intersection of global cuisines and anti-inflammatory foods—legumes, whole grains, cruciferous vegetables, and anti-inflammatory superstars—is huge, and this selection of main dish recipes is only a tiny subset of the possibilities. Whole grain pastas serve as a filling and tasty bed for all sorts of sauces and toppings, from a creamy lemon sauce to broiled cherry tomatoes with garlic. Curries and stir-fries served with rice or other grains bring joyous combinations of spices and flavors to our plates and palates. Warming casseroles like Baked Penne with Bell Peppers and Ricotta (page 222) are the ultimate in comfort foods. Or start with Bell Pepper and Mushroom Enchiladas (page 205) or Bell Pepper and Soy Curl Fajitas (page 202).

These recipes can provide templates for all sorts of variations that suit your palate. You can switch out the vegetables in the Kung Pao Soy Curls (page 210) or create your own unique Vegetable Tikka Masala Curry (page 213) with your favorite vegetable combination.

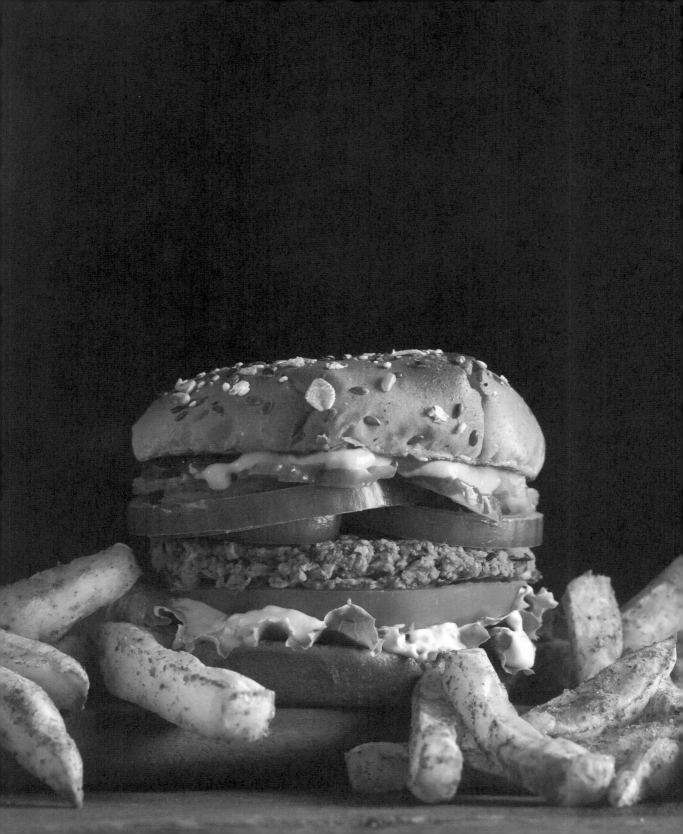

Black Bean Burgers

Makes 10–12 burger patties

These burgers have a firm, chewy texture and a savory mélange of flavors with smoked paprika undertones. The burgers are baked rather than panfried, which not only saves on oil but eliminates the time you'd have to spend standing at the stove. You can replace the beans, spices, and vegetables in this recipe with other choices and get creative with the toppings. These burgers have significantly less fat, calories, and sodium than most commercial burgers.

Preheat the oven to 425°F. Line a large sheet pan with parchment paper or a silicone mat.

Prep the chia seeds. In a small bowl, fork-whisk the following ingredients together and let them sit while you prepare the other ingredients. The mixture will be very thick.

> 1 tablespoon chia seeds, ground in a small blender, coffee grinder, or spice grinder
> ¼ cup water

Sauté the vegetables. In a skillet, water sauté the following ingredients until the onion is tender and transparent and any liquid released by the mushrooms has evaporated, 8 to 10 minutes.

> ½ cup red, yellow, or white onion, chopped
> 1 cup (4 small) white button or cremini mushrooms, chopped
> ½ cup celery, chopped
> ½ cup red bell pepper, chopped
> 1 clove garlic, finely chopped

Combine and bake. Add the following ingredients to a food processor and pulse with the following ingredients until nicely combined but still chunky.

> The sautéed vegetables
> The chia seed mixture
> 1 (15-ounce) can black beans, drained and rinsed
> 1 cup dried whole grain breadcrumbs or quick-cooking rolled oats
> ½ cup well-chopped walnuts
> 1 tablespoon ketchup
> 1 tablespoon regular or Dijon mustard
> 2 teaspoons soy sauce or tamari

(Continued on next page)

2 teaspoons Montreal steak seasoning or combination of other spices

1 teaspoon Italian seasoning

¾ teaspoon smoked paprika

Form 3- to 4-inch fairly thin patties with your hands and lay the patties on the lined pan. Bake for 12 minutes, then flip them over and bake 8 to 10 minutes more or until the patties are firm with brown surfaces.

Serve on English muffins, whole grain burger buns, or other bread with your favorite burger toppings. The patties will keep in the refrigerator for about a week. They also freeze well.

Stuffed Bell Pepper Rings

Makes 6 servings

Traditional stuffed bell peppers are tasty but the ratio of filling to pepper isn't optimal in my opinion (too much pepper!) so I experimented to find a solution. I ended up cutting each pepper into thick rings, stuffing them with a thick rice mixture, and roasting them on a sheet pan. Topped with a sauce, these stuffed rings taste and look great. They make a great choice for a holiday or other special occasion.

Preheat the oven to 400°F. Line two sheet pans with parchment paper (do not use a silicone mat because the rings tend to stick to the mat).

Make the white sauce. Put the following ingredients in a small or regular blender and blend them until completely smooth.

- **1¼ cups water**
- **1 cup tofu**
- **2 tablespoons cornstarch**
- **2 tablespoons nutritional yeast**
- **1 teaspoon lemon zest**
- **1 teaspoon onion powder**
- **1 teaspoon garlic powder**
- **1 teaspoon salt (or to taste)**
- **½ teaspoon paprika**
- **Freshly ground black pepper to taste**

In a medium saucepan over medium heat, cook the mixture, uncovered, and stir constantly until the sauce is thickened, about 3 minutes. It will be very thick. Set aside.

Make the rice. Cook the rice according to the "Whole Grains Cooking Guide" on page 43. Set aside.

- **1¼ cups uncooked brown rice**

Complete the stuffing. Stir together the following ingredients in a large bowl.

- **The thick white sauce**
- **The rice**
- **1 cup cooked vegetables (e.g., broccoli, cauliflower, peas, corn, carrots, asparagus), chopped**
- **¼ cup fresh parsley, well chopped**

(Continued on page 201)

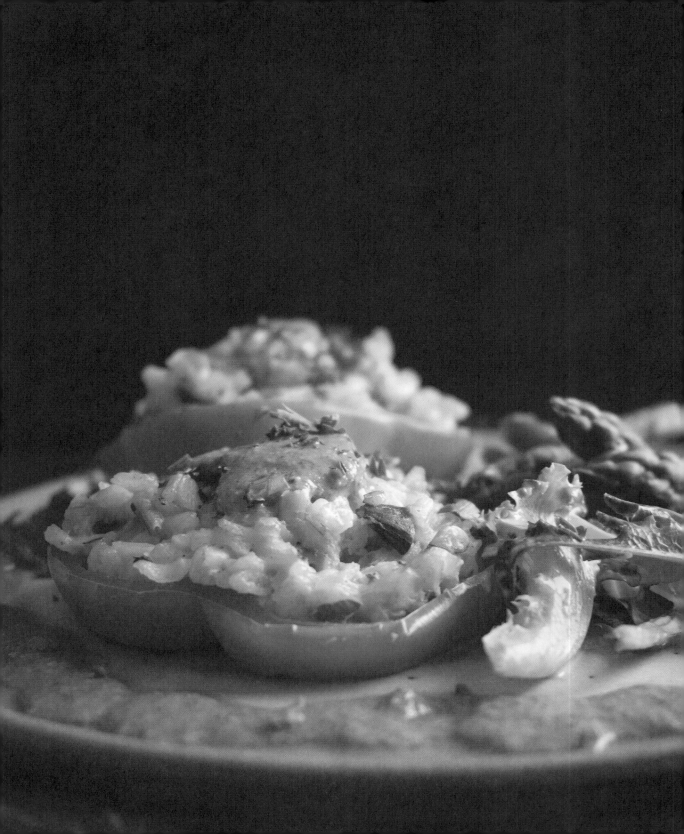

Complete the dish and bake. Cut the top off each pepper and carefully remove the seeds. Slice each pepper horizontally into ½-inch rings (1 pepper typically yields 4 to 5 rings). If the bottom rings don't sit flat, cut a little off the undersides. Lay the rings flat on the two sheet pans.

4 red bell peppers

Spoon a mound of the mixture into each pepper ring, pushing it all the way into the sides of the pepper ring. Cover with foil (no need to tuck in the foil on the sides). Bake for 30 minutes, then uncover and bake for 5 minutes more, until the peppers are tender and the filling is just golden.

They are ready to serve. I recommend serving them with a sauce or gravy. (See the "Sauces" category on graciousvegan.com for recipes or use marinara or other sauce.)

The stuffed rings will last about a week in the refrigerator. They freeze well.

Bell Pepper and Soy Curl Fajitas

Makes 4–5 servings

These fajitas boast layers of flavor and texture. Roasting brings out the best of all the ingredients, including bell peppers, soy curls, onions, tomatoes, and zucchinis. If you haven't tried soy curls yet (a healthy protein made from one ingredient: whole soybeans), this would be a great recipe to start with—you simply reconstitute them in broth and then use them like you would use cooked chicken pieces. You can control the level of spicy heat in these fajitas and decide on the types of wraps and toppings you like best.

Preheat the oven to 425°F. Line two sheet pans with parchment paper or silicone mats.

Reconstitute the soy curls. Add the dried soy curls to a medium bowl and cover them with the broth. Let them soak for about 10 minutes until the soy curls have softened. Once softened, reserve ¼ cup broth and drain the rest. Squeeze the soy curls to get out the excess broth. Set aside.

> **1 rounded cup dried soy curls**
> **1 cup vegetable broth**

Make the coating. In a bowl or jar, mix the following ingredients together.

> **¼ cup leftover broth from soaking the soy curls**
> **2 tablespoons tahini**
> **2 teaspoons chili powder**
> **1 teaspoon Mexican oregano or oregano**
> **1 teaspoon cumin**
> **1 teaspoon smoked paprika**
> **¾ teaspoon salt (or to taste)**
> **¼ teaspoon chipotle chili powder or cayenne pepper or red pepper flakes**

Assemble the mixture and roast. In a large bowl, toss the following ingredients together until all the soy curls and vegetables are coated.

> **The reconstituted soy curls**
> **The coating mixture**
> **3 red bell peppers, sliced**
> **2 Roma tomatoes, diced**
> **2 small zucchinis, sliced into ½-inch rings**
> **1 medium red, yellow, or white onion, thinly sliced or diced**
> **¼ cup fresh cilantro, chopped**

(Continued on page 204)

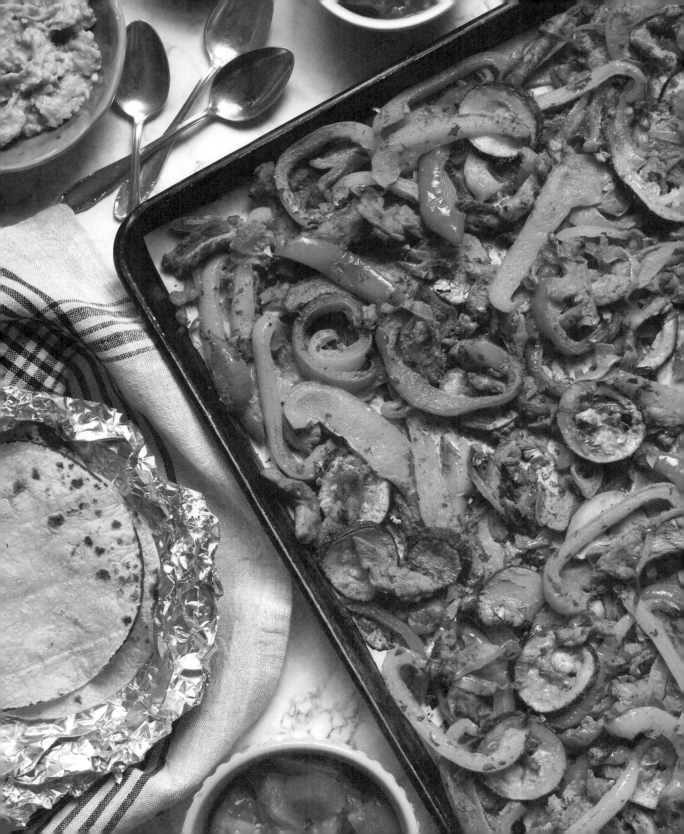

Divide the mixture onto the two sheet pans and spread out the contents into a single layer. Roast for 15 minutes, then stir and flip the vegetables. Roast for 15 more minutes, until the vegetables are tender, the liquid is evaporated, and the edges of some of the vegetables and soy curls are brown. Serve the mixture with tortillas and one or more of the following toppings.

Heated corn or whole wheat flour tortillas

Vegan crema or sour cream (see graciousvegan.com for recipes)

Guacamole (see graciousvegan.com for recipe)

Sliced green onions

Salsa

More chopped cilantro

The fajitas will keep in the refrigerator for about a week. They do not freeze well.

Bell Pepper and Mushroom Enchiladas

Makes 8 servings

I grew up in Southern California but didn't know where to find authentic Mexican food until I was older. I love all the new tastes and dishes available to us now, and I've moved way beyond the ground beef filling my mom used for everything. For this recipe I use mushrooms, onions, bell peppers, corn, and spices for the filling, with a little tofu to bind them together. If you prefer not to roll your enchiladas, you can stack them or make an enchilada casserole.

Preheat the oven to 375°F. Choose 1 large or 2 medium rectangular glass or ceramic casserole dishes.

Make the filling. Water sauté the following ingredients in a large skillet or Dutch oven until the vegetables are tender and all the liquid released by the mushrooms is evaporated, 10 to 15 minutes.

> **8 ounces white button or cremini mushrooms, diced**
> **1 small red, yellow, or white onion, diced (about 1 cup)**
> **1 small or ½ large red bell pepper, diced**
> **1 small or ½ large green bell pepper, diced**

After the vegetables are tender, add the corn and cook for a few minutes to incorporate it. Take the pan off the heat.

> **1 cup fresh, canned, or frozen corn**

Separately, in a small bowl whisk the following ingredients together until smooth.

> **½ cup silken tofu**
> **2 tablespoons nutritional yeast**
> **1 teaspoon chili powder**
> **1 teaspoon smoked paprika**
> **½ teaspoon salt (or to taste)**

Stir the tofu mixture into the sautéed vegetables for your filling.

Assemble the enchiladas and bake. If your corn tortillas are not soft and pliable, stack 5 to 6 of them at a time on a plate, cover them, and microwave them for about 20 seconds to soften them.

> **16–20 corn tortillas**

(Continued on page 207)

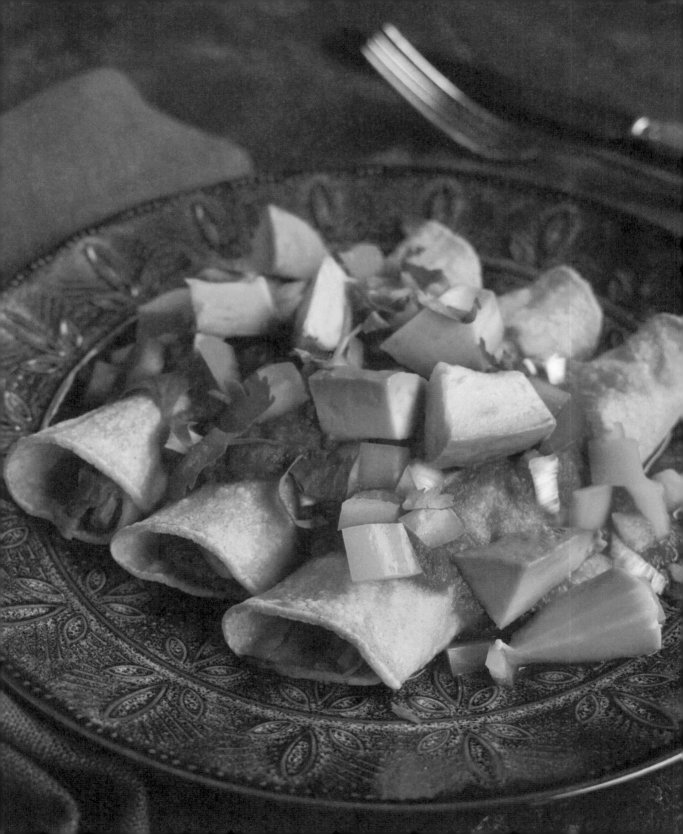

Lay the first tortilla on a cutting board or plate. Spoon 3 to 4 tablespoons of filling on one side of the circle, then roll up the tortilla. Place the enchilada at the end of the casserole dish. Continue with the rest of the tortillas and filling. Cover the casserole tightly with foil and bake for 20 to 25 minutes. You should hear some sizzling, which tells you they're baked through.

To serve the enchiladas, scoop 1 to 3 enchiladas onto the first plate and top with warmed enchilada sauce. Repeat for the remaining servings.

3 cups enchilada sauce of your choice (see graciousvegan.com for Classic Red Enchilada Sauce)

Top the enchiladas with one or more of the following toppings.

Vegan crema or sour cream (see graciousvegan.com for recipes)
Sliced green onions
Diced red onions
Diced tomatoes

The enchiladas will last about a week in the refrigerator. They can also be frozen.

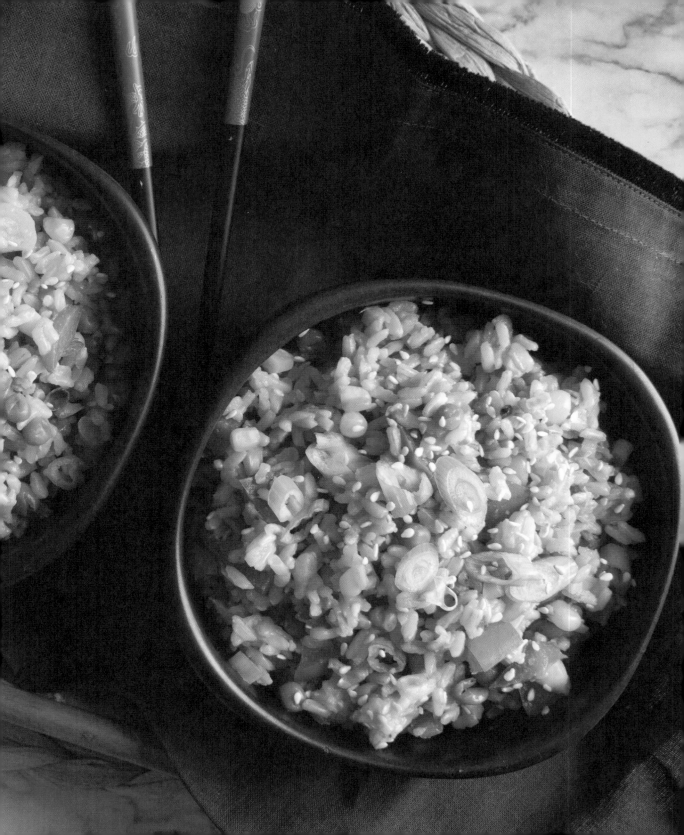

Vegetable Not-Fried Rice

Makes 4 servings

This recipe has traveled a long road. It started with my husband complaining about "rice that sticks together." Reading up on how traditional fried rice is made, I found out that experienced fried rice chefs start with cold rice, which doesn't stick or clump nearly as much as just-cooked rice. I also experimented with roasted sesame paste instead of oil, and soon the whole thing came together.

Prep the sesame paste. Whisk the roasted sesame paste or tahini with about 1 tablespoon of the soy sauce in a small bowl, then slowly whisk the remaining soy sauce into the mixture. Set aside.

1 tablespoon Chinese roasted sesame paste (see box on page 131) or tahini
¼ cup soy sauce or tamari, divided

Make the dish. Water sauté the following ingredients in a large skillet, Dutch oven, or other large pan for a few minutes until the red pepper pieces are just tender.

½ red bell pepper, deseeded and diced
The white parts of 4 green onions, sliced (see green parts used in the last step)
1½ tablespoons fresh ginger, finely chopped
2 teaspoons garlic, finely chopped

Add in the following ingredients and stir well to combine, then cook an additional 3 to 5 minutes until heated through.

4 cups cold cooked brown rice
1–2 cups baked or broiled tofu, tempeh, or seitan (optional)
½ cup fresh or frozen and thawed corn kernels
½ cup fresh or frozen and thawed peas
The sesame paste mixture

Add in the following ingredients and stir to combine.

The green parts of 4 green onions, sliced
⅛ cup or more lightly toasted sesame seeds, walnuts, cashews, pine nuts, almonds, or peanuts

The dish is ready to serve. It will keep in the refrigerator for about a week. It does not freeze well.

Kung Pao Soy Curls

Makes 4 servings

Soy curls are a great substitute for chicken in this recipe. They come out chewy, roasted on the outside, soft on the inside, and they soak up the wonderful flavors of the sauce. While the three-stage roasting method looks complicated at first, once you've worked through it, you'll find that it's easy and it avoids multiple pots and pans. You can substitute other vegetables for the red pepper and broccoli, although both are anti-inflammatory superstars. The peanuts and fresh cilantro at the end make this dish sing.

Preheat the oven to 425°F. Line a sheet pan with parchment paper or a silicone mat.

Reconstitute the soy curls. Add the dried soy curls to a medium bowl and cover with the broth. Let soak for about 10 minutes until the soy curls have softened. Once softened, drain the broth and squeeze the soy curls to get out the excess broth. Set aside.

> **1 rounded cup dried soy curls**
> **1 cup warm vegetable broth**

Make the sauce. Blend together the following ingredients in a blender until smooth.

> **4 cloves garlic, finely chopped**
> **½ cup vegetable broth**
> **¼ cup soy sauce or tamari**
> **2 tablespoons Chinese roasted sesame paste (see box on page 131) or sesame oil**
> **2 tablespoons rice vinegar**
> **2 tablespoons maple syrup**
> **1½ tablespoons peanut butter**
> **2 teaspoons fresh ginger, finely chopped**
> **Large pinch Chinese five spice powder**
> **¾ teaspoon chili garlic sauce or your choice of red pepper flakes, sriracha, or other chili**

Roast stage 1. Put the soy curls and sauce in a medium bowl and toss to coat the soy curls. Use a slotted spoon to transfer the curls to the prepared sheet pan. Arrange in a single layer and roast for 8 minutes.

While the soy curls are roasting, toss the red pepper and broccoli in the sauce in the same bowl.

> **1 red bell pepper, cut into bite-size pieces**
> **1 head broccoli, cut into florets (3–4 cups)**

(Continued on page 212)

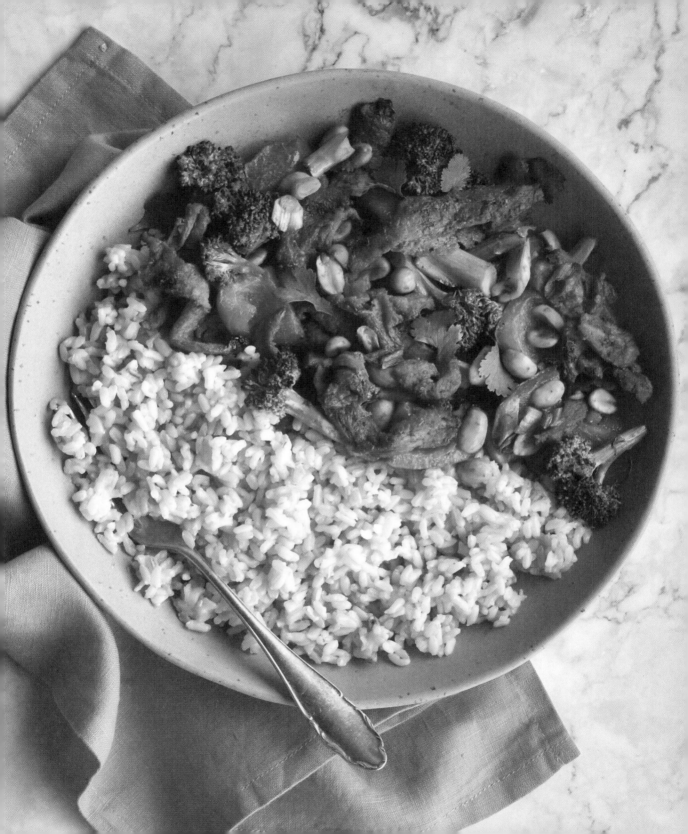

Roast stage 2. Take the soy curls out of the oven, flip them over, and use a slotted spoon to add the red pepper and broccoli to the pan. Preserve as much sauce as possible in the bowl. Spread the vegetables across the sheet pan around the soy curls. Roast another 10 minutes.

Roast stage 3. Remove the pan from the oven and scatter the peanuts and green onions over the pan.

⅓ cup roasted peanuts, whole or chopped
3 green onions, thinly sliced

Continue cooking until the soy curls are browned and the vegetables are tender, about 5 more minutes.

Finish the sauce and serve. Heat the remaining sauce in the microwave or in a saucepan so it's ready to serve. Remove the pan from the oven, sprinkle the cilantro on top, and serve the mixture with rice or quinoa and the sauce.

1 handful fresh cilantro leaves, roughly chopped
Cooked brown rice or quinoa

The mixture will last about a week in the refrigerator. It does not freeze well.

Vegetable Tikka Masala Curry

Makes 5 servings

Curry sauces are so helpful to a plant-based lifestyle. You can use them in a bowl with grains and vegetables, on baked potatoes, and with burgers or patties or even pasta. Tikka masala is a tomato and cream sauce often made with heavy cream or yogurt. Here I use cashews and blend them with water for a smooth milk that thickens once it's stirred into the wonderfully spiced tomato base. You can make it as mild or spicy as you like. I often serve soy curls and vegetables with this sauce on top of rice.

Make the cashew milk. Soak the cashews in water for 2 hours or pour boiling water over them, cover, let them soak for about 20 minutes, then drain them.

½ cup raw cashews

Put the cashews in a blender with the water. Blend on high for 30 seconds or longer, until the cashews are dissolved. Set aside.

¾ cup water

Make the sauce. Water sauté the following ingredients together in a large saucepan or skillet until the onion is tender and transparent, 8 to 10 minutes.

½ cup red, yellow, or white onion, diced
2 cloves garlic, finely chopped
1 teaspoon fresh ginger, finely chopped

Add in the following ingredients and cook, stirring constantly, for about 4 minutes, until the mixture is fragrant.

2 tablespoons tomato paste
1 teaspoon turmeric
1 teaspoon cumin
1 teaspoon coriander
¾ teaspoon garam masala
½ teaspoon salt (or to taste)
½ teaspoon freshly ground black pepper (or more to taste)
¼ teaspoon red pepper flakes or Kashmiri chili powder (or more to taste)
¼ teaspoon cardamom

(Continued on page 215)

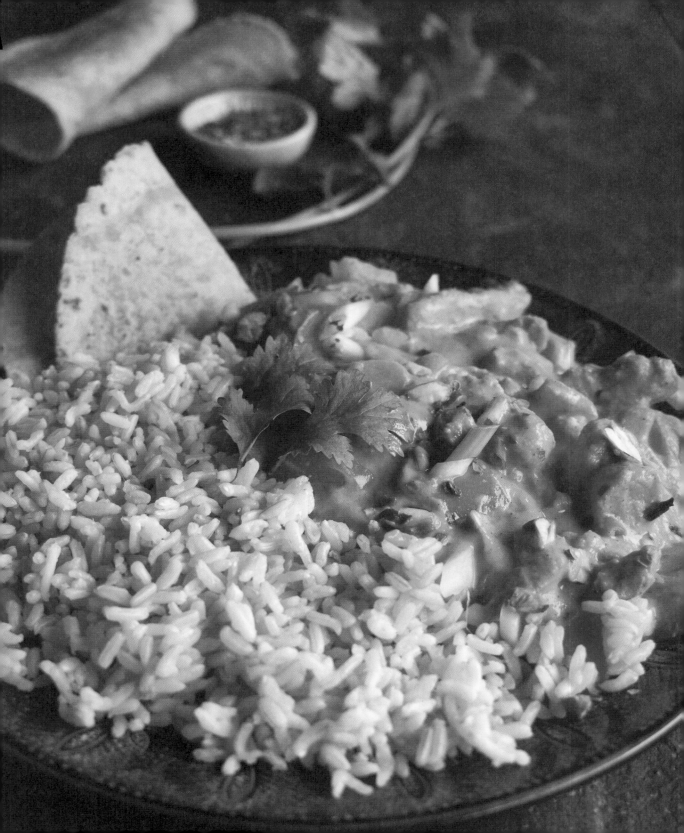

Add in the diced tomatoes, increase the heat, bring the mixture to a boil, then reduce the heat. Simmer with the lid ajar, stirring occasionally, for about 10 minutes, adding a little water if it gets too dry.

1 (15-ounce) can fire-roasted or plain diced tomatoes

Add in the following ingredients and simmer for 5 minutes, stirring often, until thick. Add water, if needed, and adjust seasonings after tasting.

The cashew milk
⅓ loosely packed cup fresh cilantro leaves and stems, chopped

Blend the sauce until smooth, if desired. I prefer to let it cool a bit and then blend it in my high-speed blender so that it is very smooth.

Create a vegetable curry. For each serving, prepare about 1 cup steamed or cooked vegetables. Stir the vegetables together with the warm curry sauce and serve with rice.

Steamed or cooked vegetables (red bell peppers, broccoli, cauliflower, peas, kale, etc.)
Cooked brown basmati- or long-grain rice

The sauce keeps in the refrigerator for about a week. The sauce freezes well.

Asparagus with Orzo and Breadcrumbs

Makes 4 servings

A favorite of my students, this recipe highlights the tartness of lemons, the boldness of fresh herbs, and the crispness of breadcrumbs. The abundant asparagus pieces shout, "It's spring!" This dish works for brunch as well as dinner, because it tastes great both at room temperature and when heated. I love it for lunch and can eat it all week long. Seek out whole wheat orzo if you have the time—you'll get the benefit of extra fiber.

Make the pasta and asparagus. Bring a medium pot of water to a boil. Add the orzo and cook until al dente according to package directions. Two minutes before the orzo is done, add in the asparagus. Drain the orzo and asparagus.

- **1 cup uncooked whole wheat orzo or other small pasta**
- **1 pound asparagus, trimmed and sliced on a diagonal (if asparagus is thick, slice about ¼-inch thick)**

Make the dressing. While the orzo and asparagus cook, in a large mixing bowl make the dressing by stirring the following ingredients together.

- **1½ tablespoons tahini**
- **1½ tablespoons water**
- **1 teaspoon lemon zest plus 3 tablespoons freshly squeezed lemon juice from 1 large lemon**
- **¼ teaspoon salt (or to taste)**
- **Freshly ground black pepper to taste**

Add the drained orzo and asparagus into the dressing and toss to coat. Set aside while you toast the breadcrumbs.

Make the breadcrumbs. In a large skillet without the heat on, add the following ingredients and stir together.

- **1 tablespoon tahini**
- **1 tablespoon water**

Add in the breadcrumbs and garlic powder, stir them into the water-tahini mixture, and season with salt and pepper.

(Continued on page 218)

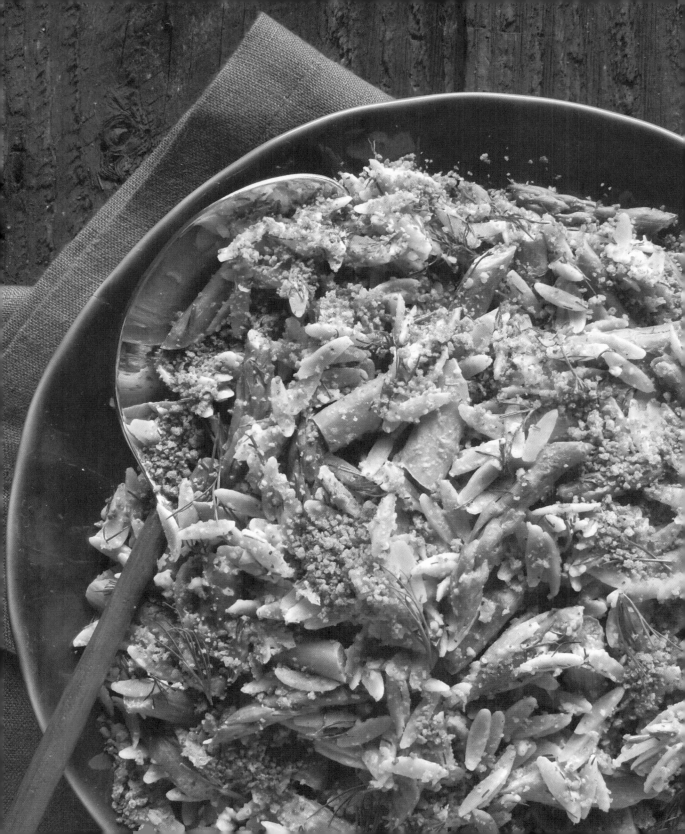

⅓ **cup dry whole wheat breadcrumbs**
¼ **teaspoon garlic powder**
Salt and pepper to taste

Start the heat on medium and cook the breadcrumbs, stirring often, until they are golden, 3 to 5 minutes, then remove from the heat.

Assemble and serve. Stir the vegan Parmesan and herbs into the dressed orzo, taste, and adjust seasoning. Top with the toasted breadcrumbs and more vegan Parmesan if you like.

¼ **cup vegan Parmesan, plus more for garnish (see graciousvegan.com for a recipe)**
½ **cup fresh dill, mint, and/or parsley leaves, chopped or torn**

Serve immediately, warm or at room temperature. The dish will keep in the refrigerator for a few days (you may need to add a little water when you warm it up). It does not freeze well.

The Plant-Based Anti-Inflammatory Cookbook

Pasta with Arugula
in a Creamy Lemon Sauce

Makes 5 servings

This lighter and anti-inflammatory version of a favorite pasta combination lets the main flavors shine through. The peppery arugula stands out well against the velvety lemon-sauce, while the broccoli and pasta provide a tasty base. In preparing this dish, have the cashew cream done before starting to cook the other elements, then aim for the pasta and broccoli to finish cooking at the same time so everything can be tossed together and served immediately.

Make the cashew cream. Soak the cashews in water for 2 hours or pour boiling water over them, cover, let them soak for about 20 minutes, then drain them.

½ cup raw cashews

Put the cashews in a blender with the water. Blend on high for 30 seconds or longer, until the cashews are dissolved. Set aside.

¾ cup water

Make the pasta. Cook the pasta in a saucepan according to package directions. When it is done to your liking, drain the pasta.

8 ounces uncooked whole grain pasta such as fusilli (spirals), penne, or other shape

Cook broccoli and complete the dish. While the pasta is cooking, cook the following ingredients in a Dutch oven or other large pot, covered, with several tablespoons of water, for 3 to 4 minutes, until tender.

1 clove garlic, finely chopped
3–4 cups broccoli florets

Add the following ingredients to the garlic and broccoli, stir together, and cook a few minutes more until the cream is thickened and the arugula has wilted. Add water if needed.

The cashew cream
5 ounces fresh baby arugula
1 cup grape or cherry tomatoes, halved
Zest and juice from 1 lemon
¾ teaspoon salt (or to taste)
Freshly ground black pepper to taste

(Continued on page 221)

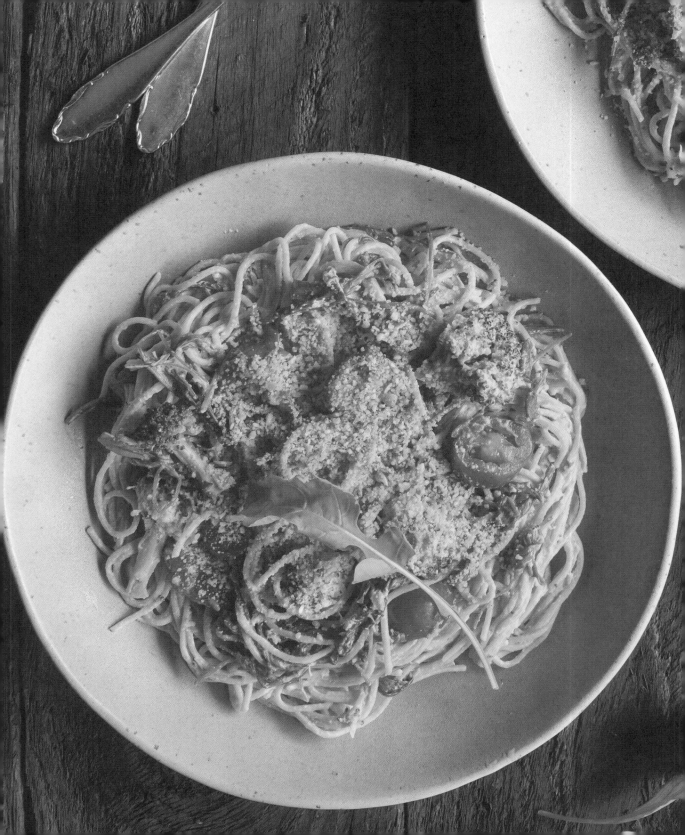

Add the pasta to the sauce, toss them together, and transfer to a serving dish or dishes. Serve with vegan Parmesan sprinkled on top.

The cooked pasta

¼–½ cup vegan Parmesan (see graciousvegan.com for a recipe)

The pasta will keep in the refrigerator for a few days, though you may have to add water when you reheat it. It does not freeze well.

Baked Penne with
Bell Peppers and Ricotta

Makes 8 servings

A hot baked pasta dish is as comforting as a blanket around your shoulders. With healthy plant-based ricotta and Parmesan cheeses we can avoid many grams of saturated fats and still enjoy the steamy, creamy, tomatoey goodness of a hot pasta bake. You can change the vegetables if bell peppers and mushrooms aren't your favorites, and you can use your favorite small pasta shape. The Italian Chopped Salad with Sun-Dried Tomato Dressing on page 94 goes well with this dish for dinner.

Preheat the oven to 425°F. Serve in an 11 × 8-inch casserole dish.

Cook the vegetables. In a large skillet, Dutch oven, or other pan, water sauté the following ingredients until the vegetables are just tender, and the liquid released by the mushrooms is evaporated, 8 to 10 minutes.

> **8 ounces white button, baby bella, or cremini mushrooms, sliced or chopped**
> **1 red bell pepper, cut into bite-sized pieces (larger than dice)**
> **3 cloves garlic, finely chopped**
> **½ teaspoon ground fennel seeds**

Cook the pasta. Separately, boil the pasta for 2 minutes less than the package instructions. When draining the pasta, reserve ⅓ cup of the pasta water.

> **8 ounces uncooked whole grain penne pasta or other shape**

Assemble and bake. In a large bowl, stir together the following ingredients.

> **The sautéed vegetables**
> **The cooked pasta**
> **The reserved pasta water**
> **2 cups marinara sauce**
> **¾ cup (about 1½ ounces) fresh basil, chopped**
> **Salt and freshly ground pepper to taste**

Spoon the mixture into the casserole dish, then spoon dollops of ricotta over the mixture and use a knife to swirl the dollops into the pasta so that they get distributed but not entirely mixed in.

(Continued on page 224)

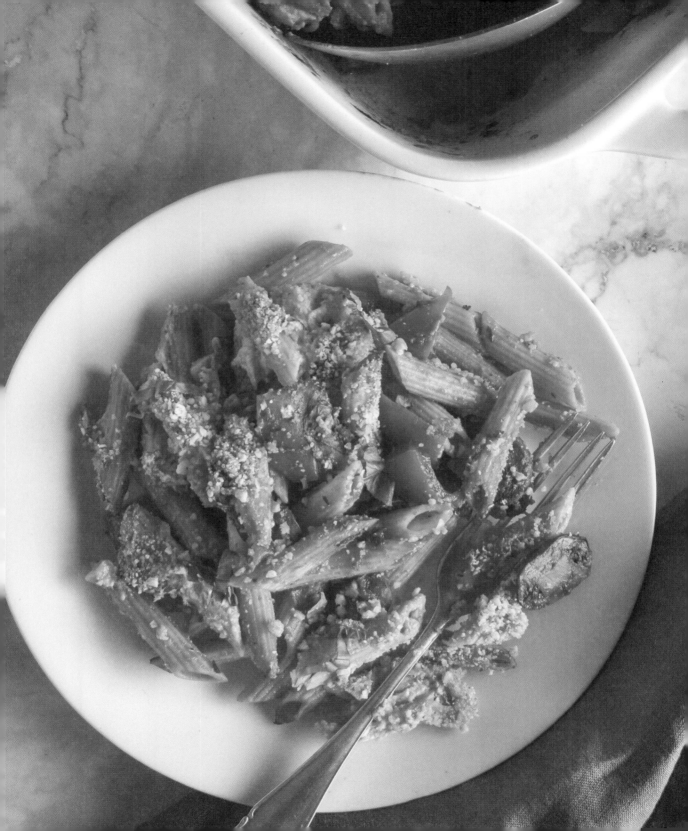

1 cup vegan ricotta cheese (if it is very thick, stir in some water or nondairy milk to achieve a texture that will let you dollop and swirl it; see graciousvegan.com for a recipe)

Sprinkle vegan Parmesan cheese over the top.

½–1 cup vegan Parmesan cheese (see graciousvegan.com for a recipe)

Bake 20 to 25 minutes or until you can hear bubbling, and the top is golden brown.

The casserole is ready to serve. It will last in the refrigerator for about a week. It can be frozen, although the top won't be as crispy, and the casserole will not be as moist.

Pasta e Fagioli

Makes 5 servings

"When the stars make you drool, like a pasta fazool / That's amore!" This dish is worth singing about! The fresh basil and spice combination of oregano, thyme, and garlic give it a classically satisfying taste. Top it with vegan Parmesan and take it to another level. Some recipes for Pasta e Fagioli make it into a stew or soup, but I prefer it as a tossed pasta dish. This dish pairs well with crusty whole grain bread and a salad such as Apple and Greens with Candied Walnuts (page 89).

Put the following ingredients in a Dutch oven or soup pot and bring to a boil. Reduce heat and simmer, partly covered, until vegetables are tender, 10 to 15 minutes.

1 small or ½ large red, yellow, or white onion, diced (about 1 cup)

3 cloves garlic, finely chopped

2 medium carrots, diced or chopped

2 celery stalks, diced or chopped

1 cup vegetable broth or water

Add in the following ingredients and simmer for another 10 to 15 minutes, partly covered.

2 (15-ounce) cans kidney beans or small red beans, drained and rinsed

1 (16-ounce) can tomato sauce

1 (15-ounce) can diced or petite-diced tomatoes

1 tablespoon tomato paste

1½ teaspoons dried oregano

¾ teaspoon dried thyme

While the sauce is cooking, cook the pasta to al dente according to package instructions; drain well and set aside.

1 cup uncooked whole grain small pasta (ditalini is my favorite, but any kind will do)

After the sauce is cooked, add the following ingredients, toss together, and serve.

The cooked pasta

⅓ cup fresh basil, chopped or sliced, or 1½ teaspoons dried basil added earlier with the other spices

½ teaspoon salt (or to taste)

(Continued on page 227)

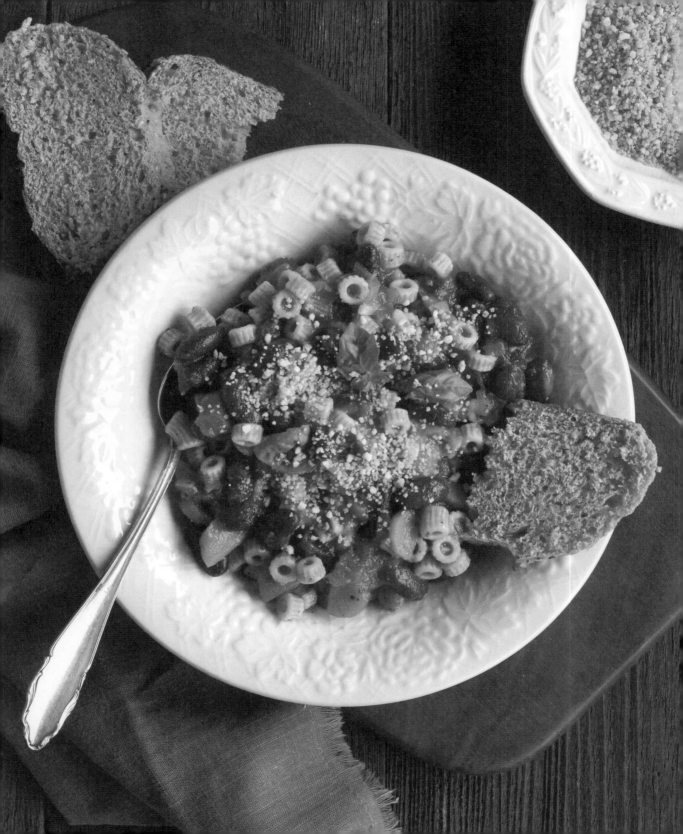

Top each serving with Parmesan cheese, if desired.

Vegan Parmesan cheese (see graciousvegan.com for a recipe)

Serve immediately. The dish will keep well in the refrigerator for about a week. It freezes well, though the pasta will absorb most of the liquid, so you will need to add in more water or tomato sauce when you warm it.

Garlicky Cherry Tomatoes with Angel Hair Pasta

Makes 4 servings

This easy recipe turns grape or cherry tomatoes into an intriguing pasta dish that will bring folks back for more. The combination of garlic, tomato juices, fresh basil, and vegan Parmesan creates a well-balanced sauce that coats angel hair pasta especially well. Using the broiler for roasting the tomatoes means less time for preheating and less heat in your kitchen on a warm evening.

Start a large pot of water to boil. Adjust oven rack to upper-middle position (about 6 inches from broiler). Use a 15 × 10-inch Pyrex pan or large rimmed baking sheet lined with foil. Turn on the broiler to high (500°F).

Spread the tomatoes on the baking sheet and sprinkle with salt. Broil the tomatoes, shaking the pan every 5 minutes or so, until the tomatoes are cracked, very soft, and shrunken, 12 to 20 minutes. They'll be blackened in places.

2 pints (20 ounces) or cherry or grape tomatoes
¼ teaspoon salt (or to taste)

Microwave the garlic cloves for 45 to 60 seconds to soften them. Then chop them. Alternatively, boil the cloves for about 2 minutes with the pasta, then fish them out of the water and chop them.

4 large or 5 small cloves garlic

Cook the pasta in the large pot of boiling water according to package directions and drain. Return the pasta to the pot.

5 ounces uncooked whole wheat angel hair pasta or thin spaghetti

Add the following ingredients to the pasta pot and toss them together with the pasta.

The tomatoes
The garlic
⅓ cup vegan Parmesan cheese (see graciousvegan.com for a recipe)
¼ packed cup fresh basil leaves, ribboned
½ teaspoon salt (or to taste)
⅛ teaspoon (or to taste) red pepper flakes
Freshly ground pepper to taste

The dish is ready to serve. The pasta will keep in the refrigerator for 3 or 4 days, although the pasta will swell and absorb any juices. The dish does not freeze well.

The Plant-Based Anti-Inflammatory Cookbook

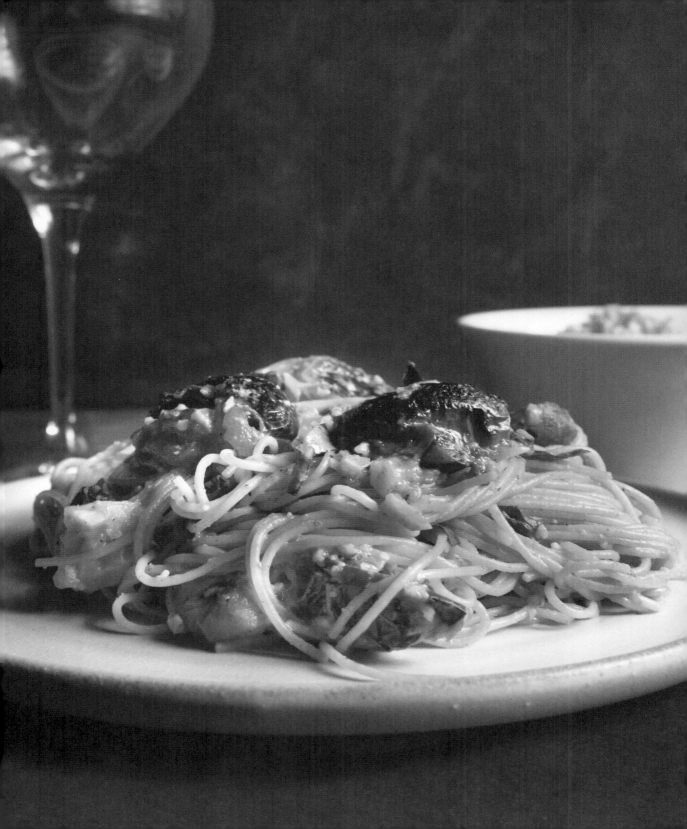

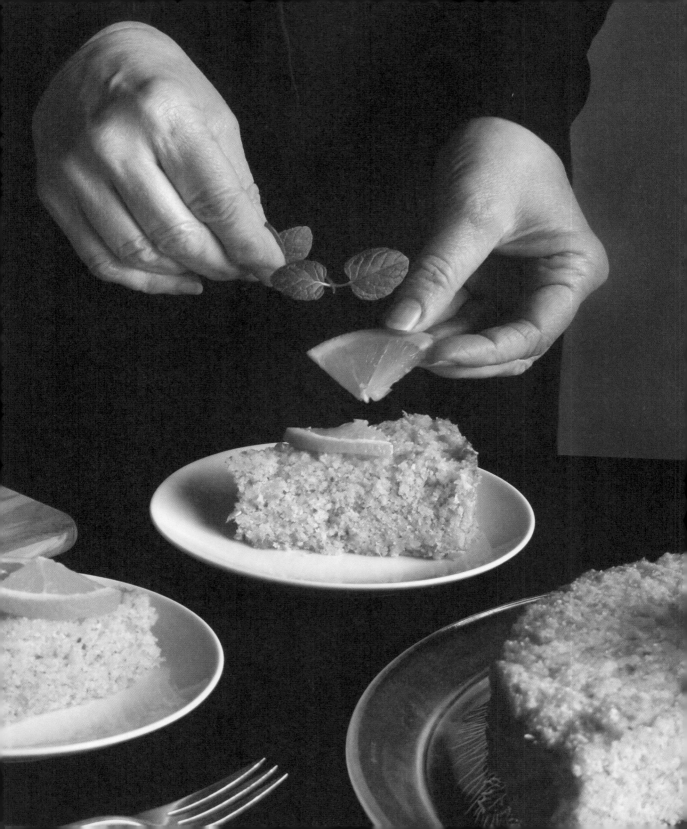

Sweets

Too many times in swanky coffee houses I've noticed that the only vegan treats they have are large, dull, cellophane-wrapped cookies full of refined flour and sugar. I wish more people understood how good healthy plant-based sweets can be.

I've tinkered my way to recipes for baked cookies, no-bake cookies, bar cookies, cakes, cheesecakes, sundaes, fruit crisps, and killer sauces, all without refined flour, sugar, eggs, or oils. It can be done!

If sugary treats have been a big part of your life, they can be very hard to give up. We sometimes don't realize how strong the little habits of our day are until we resolve to stop them. I hope that one or more of these healthy, anti-inflammatory sweets can replace your habits with better ones and help you bring down the amount of pro-inflammatory foods in your diet.

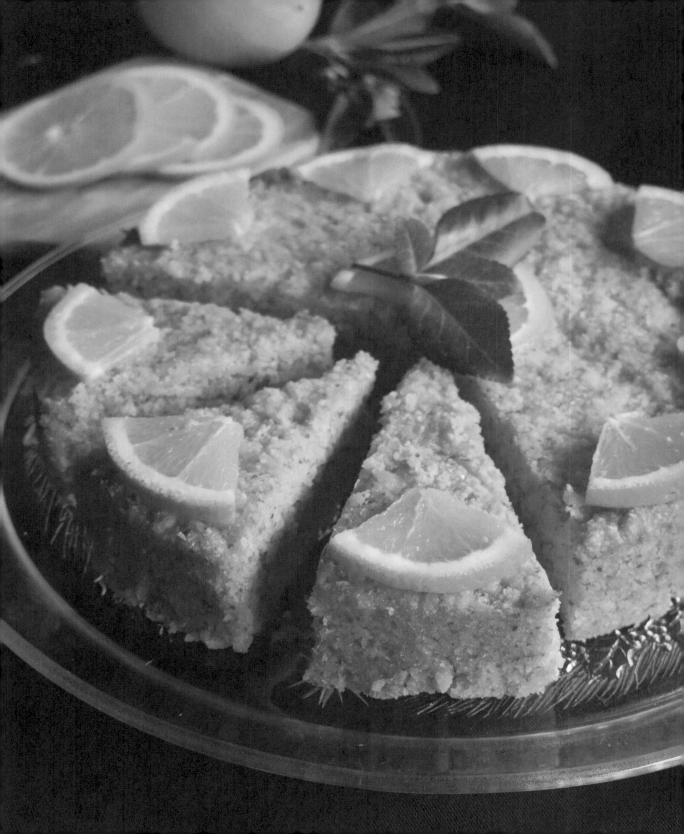

Orange-Ginger Polenta Cake

Makes 1 (9-inch) round cake or 2 (8-inch) round layers (not as tall as the 9-inch cake)

Talk about low food waste! This cake uses two whole oranges, including the rind. Boiling oranges removes the bitterness and makes the oranges easy to blend into a puree that substitutes well for oil and lends a complex orange flavor to the cake. Dense and moist, this cake tastes great chilled, at room temperature, or warm. It also goes well with many different toppings besides the ones listed below—try it with berries, cherries, a compote, or sugar-free marmalade. Oranges are now available year-round, but this cake makes a dramatic dessert for the winter holidays.

Boil the oranges. In a large saucepan, cover the oranges with water.

   2 whole navel oranges, unpeeled

Cover the pan, bring to a boil, then reduce the heat to a simmer and simmer the oranges for 45 minutes. When they are done, remove the oranges and let them cool a bit (about 15 minutes).

Once the oranges have cooled, cut each into 8 to 12 chunks (leaving the peel on).

Make the cake. Preheat the oven to 375°F. Line 1 (9-inch) round cake pan or 2 (8-inch) pans with parchment paper.

Blend the following ingredients together in a blender until the oranges are partially pureed. (It's good to leave some small chunks of orange.) Set aside.

   The chunks of 2 boiled oranges
   1 cup maple syrup
   ½ cup applesauce
   ¼ cup plain or vanilla plant-based yogurt or nondairy milk
   2–3 tablespoons fresh ginger, finely chopped

Separately, in a medium mixing bowl stir or whisk together the following ingredients.

   1½ cups polenta or cornmeal (see box on page 160)
   1¼ cups almond flour or well-ground almonds
   1½ teaspoons baking powder

Pour the blended mixture into the dry mixture and stir gently until everything is combined. Pour the batter into the prepared cake pan(s) and bake for 45 to 55 minutes or until the edges are dark golden. The top may show some cracks, which is fine.

(Continued on next page)

Remove the cake(s) from the oven and let the cake(s) cool in the pan completely on a cooling rack. When cool, remove the cake(s) from the pan(s). Serve with cream and orange slices if desired.

Ginger-Infused Cream Topping (page 264)
Thin orange slices

The cake will last 4 to 5 days in the refrigerator, although it dries out a bit. It can be frozen.

Year-Round Fruitcake

Makes 4 (8 × 4-inch) loaves or can be made in other pans

Bursting with fruit and nuts, this dense fruitcake tastes great any time of year. Most traditional fruitcakes require eggs (lots of them), sugar, candied fruits, and butter. This version avoids those pro-inflammatory ingredients in favor of chia seeds, date syrup, dried fruit, and prune puree. You can customize your fruitcake with your favorite nuts and dried fruits—go tropical with pineapple, mango, coconut, banana, and macadamia nuts, for example. I love to make small loaves to give away, as well as a larger loaf or two that I can chisel away at myself.

Preheat the oven to 275°F.

Prep the pans. To serve as a dessert cake, plan on using about half the batter in an 8- or 9-inch round cake pan or all the batter in 4 (8 × 4-inch) bread pans, multiple mini loaf pans, tube pans, or even cupcake molds. Line pans with parchment paper or muffin paper cups.

Prep the fruit. You'll need about 1 pound of dried fruit. Chop the fruit into small pieces with a heavy, sharp knife (this helps avoid a crumbly cake). Feel free to substitute other dried fruit or change the amounts to total 1 pound. In my experience, dried apples lend a key flavor.

- **6 ounces dried apples**
- **4 ounces dried pineapple**
- **4 ounces date bits**
- **4 ounces dried apricots**
- **4 ounces raisins or currants**
- **4 ounces dried cranberries**
- **4 ounces dried cherries**

Prep the nuts. Chop the nuts into small pieces (again, this helps avoid a crumbly cake).

- **1 pound walnuts, pecans, or other nuts**

Make the chia mixture. In a small bowl, fork-whisk the following ingredients together. The mixture will be very thick. Set aside.

- **1¼ cups warm water**
- **¼ cup chia seeds, ground in a small blender, coffee grinder, or spice grinder**

(Continued on page 237)

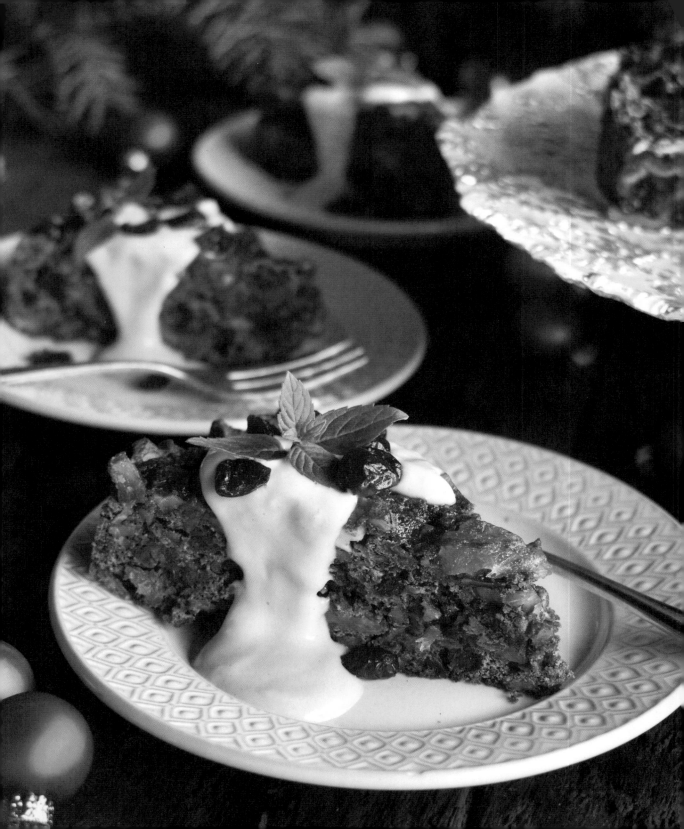

Mix the dry ingredients. Sift the following ingredients together in a medium bowl. Set aside.

3 cups whole wheat pastry flour
1½ tablespoons baking powder
2½ teaspoons cinnamon
2 teaspoons cloves
2 teaspoons allspice
2 teaspoons nutmeg
1 teaspoon mace
½ teaspoon salt (or to taste)

Mix the wet ingredients. In a separate bowl, whisk or stir the following ingredients together.

1½ cups date syrup or maple syrup
½ cup prune paste (see Mary McDougall's recipe on drmcdougall.com or use prune baby food)
½ cup unsweetened nondairy milk
2 teaspoons vanilla extract or vanilla powder

Put it all together. Add the chia egg mixture to the wet ingredients and stir or whisk by hand to combine well. Add half the dry ingredients to the wet ingredients. Stir to incorporate them without over-beating. Repeat with the second half of the dry ingredients. Add the fruit and nuts and use a wooden spoon (or, if needed, your hands) to mix it all up. Spoon the batter into the prepared pans, pressing down firmly to fill in the corners. You can fill the pans almost to the brim because the cake will rise only slightly.

Bake. Place the pans in the middle or lower third of the oven for 1 to 2 hours, until a knife or toothpick comes out clean, the top is a shade darker, and the fruit on top starts to change to darker colors (the dried apples are an especially good indication of this). Timing is extremely variable. Test each cake separately and take it out as soon as your tester comes out clean. My experience has been that almost any size takes at least an hour. If you have a hot oven, the time may be shorter.

When the cakes are done, let them cool on racks in their pans. When they are cool, use a plastic knife to loosen any stuck spots. Remove them from the pans and store in airtight wrapping in the refrigerator. The cakes last at least a month in the refrigerator and can be frozen for about a month. They tend to dry out quicker than traditional fruitcake because of the lack of oil.

Raspberry Cheesecake with Raspberry Sauce

Makes 1 (8–8½-inch) cheesecake

Cheesecakes should above all be rich and creamy. Done! This recipe's cashew-based filling balances perfectly with the sharp taste of the raspberries. I couldn't decide between hiding the raspberries inside the cheesecake or topping it with a raspberry sauce, so I did both. You can use fresh or frozen raspberries or substitute other berries like blueberries and blackberries. In Portland, high summer brings as many wild blackberries as you can pick—their gargantuan canes pop up all over the place. It's critical to blend the soaked cashews until they are completely smooth.

Soak the cashews. Soak the cashews in water for 2 hours or pour boiling water over them, cover, let them soak for about 20 minutes, then drain them. Set aside.

> **1¾ cups raw cashews**

Make the crust. Process the following ingredients in a food processor until they start to clump. Add additional teaspoons of water if the mixture isn't clumping.

> **⅓ cup sliced or slivered almonds**
> **⅓ cup walnuts**
> **⅓ cup old fashioned oats**
> **4 pitted Medjool dates, cut into chunks (about ⅓ cup)**
> **3 tablespoons unsweetened shredded coconut**
> **1 teaspoon vanilla extract or vanilla powder**
> **1 teaspoon water**

Press the mixture into the bottom of an 8- or 8½-inch springform pan.

Make the filling. Put the following ingredients together in a blender. Blend on high for 30 seconds or longer, until the cashews are dissolved.

> **The soaked and drained cashews**
> **⅓ cup maple syrup**
> **⅓ cup freshly squeezed lemon juice from 2 medium lemons**
> **Zest from 1 medium lemon**
> **1½ teaspoons vanilla extract or vanilla powder**

(Continued on page 240)

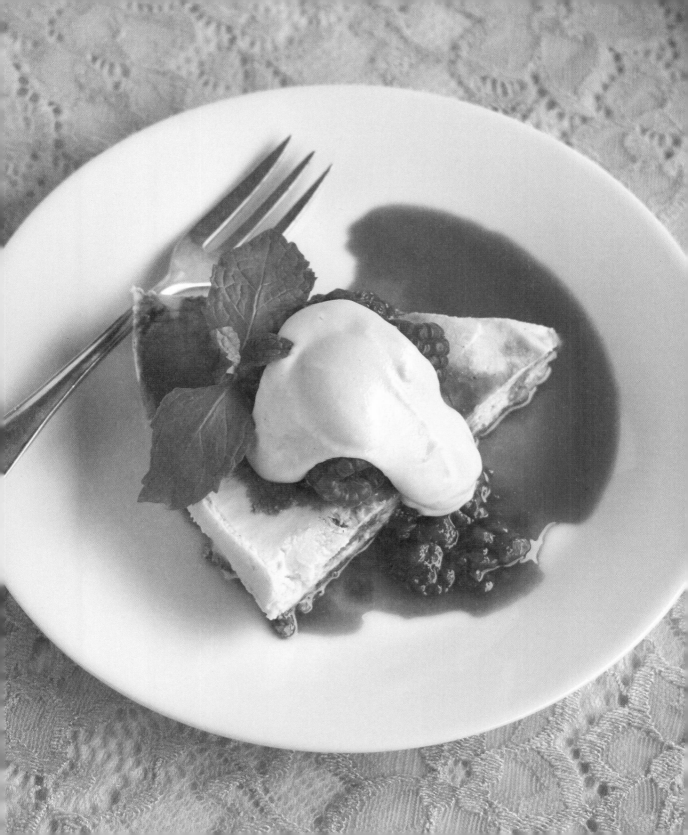

Complete the cheesecake. Add a single layer of berries on top of the crust.

1½ cups fresh or frozen raspberries

Gently dollop the filling on top of the raspberries and nudge the filling into the crevices around the berries. Use a spatula to level off the surface. Freeze the cheesecake for an hour, then serve, or leave it in the freezer for later. If it is completely frozen, take it out of the freezer and let it sit on the counter at room temperature for 30 to 60 minutes. Serve with raspberry sauce.

Chunky Raspberry Sauce (see below)

The cheesecake will last in the freezer for 2 to 3 months.

Chunky Raspberry Sauce

Stir together the following ingredients in a medium saucepan.

2 cups fresh raspberries or 10–12 ounces frozen raspberries
¼ cup water
¼ cup maple syrup

Bring the mixture to a boil, then lower the heat and simmer, uncovered, for 4 to 6 minutes, stirring occasionally, until the sauce is thicker than when it started (it will still be a bit thin but will thicken as it cools).

Stir in the vanilla.

2 teaspoons vanilla extract or vanilla powder

Transfer the sauce into a container and chill it for about an hour. It is ready to serve. It will last in the refrigerator for about a week and can be frozen.

Cherry Nice Cream
with Raw Brownie Bits

Makes about 2 cups nice cream

There's just something about the combination of cherries and chocolate. In this recipe, blending frozen cherries with bananas (full of sweetness and lightness) yields a soft, smooth base. Folding in pieces of raw brownies takes the dessert to a whole new level. You can make this nice cream during cherry season and top it with fresh cherries or use frozen cherries any time of year. I use a food processor for making nice cream, but high-speed blenders work just as well. Both methods usually require stops, starts, and wipe-downs, and blenders often need a bit more liquid.

Make the raw brownies. Note that this brownie recipe makes more than you will need for the dessert. You'll just have to eat the rest (!). Or you can cut this brownie recipe in half and make just enough for the dessert.

Line a loaf pan with parchment or wax paper. Add the dates to the food processor and blend them until you see a smooth paste (the mixture may form into a ball).

> **7 (¾ cup) pitted Medjool dates**

Add in the following ingredients and process until well combined.

> **¼ cup almond flour**
> **¼ cup cocoa powder**
> **1 teaspoon vanilla extract or vanilla powder**

Add in the following ingredients and process until the mixture is combined and you can still see tiny pieces of pecans.

> **¾ cup roasted pecans**
> **1½ tablespoons maple syrup**

Transfer the mixture to the pan and press down well. Refrigerate for at least an hour, but preferably 2 hours.

Make the nice cream. Add the following ingredients to a food processor or blender and process/blend them until you get a mixture that looks like smooth soft serve ice cream. You may have to stop the machine once or twice to wipe down the sides, but don't worry, it will get there within a few minutes.

(Continued on page 243)

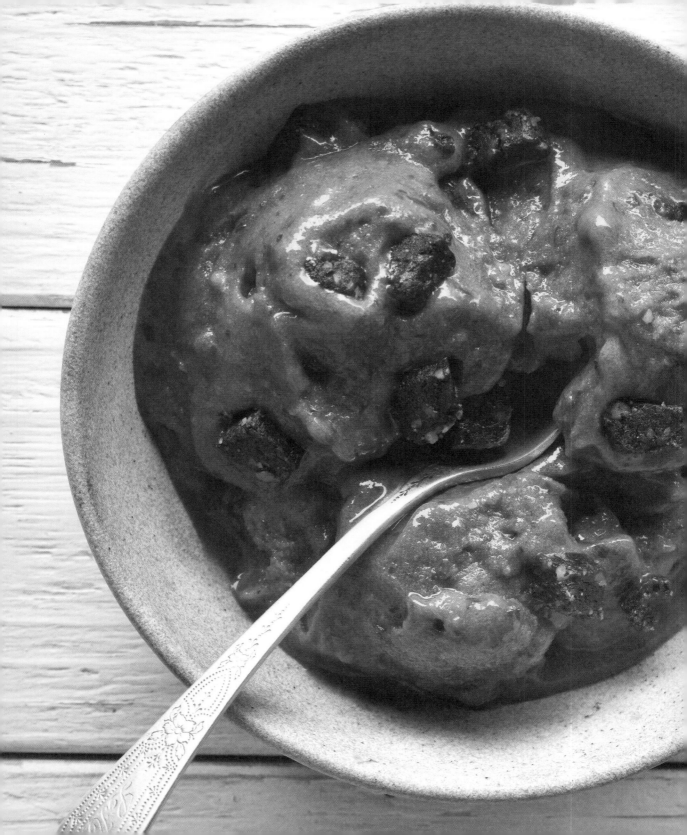

1½ cups frozen cherries, pitted and halved

1 frozen banana, sliced

¼ cup nondairy milk

1 teaspoon vanilla extract or vanilla powder

By hand, stir in small cubes of the raw brownies. Serve the nice cream immediately or freeze it. If you hard-freeze it, take it out of the freezer 45 to 60 minutes before serving or soften it in the microwave for 20 to 30 seconds, then in 15-second increments between stirrings as needed. It will keep about a month in the freezer.

Walnut and Date Caramel Tart

Makes 8 servings

Perfect for a special occasion, potluck, or dinner party, this lovely tart starts with an almost buttery crust bursting with walnuts and oats. A layer of blended dates, almond butter, and vanilla forms the caramel filling, and chocolate sauce on top pulls it all together. To take it up one more notch, you can dollop each piece with cream topping. If you don't have a springform pan, you can use a pie plate.

Preheat the oven to 350°F. Use an 8-inch springform pan.

Toast the nuts. Spread walnuts in a single layer on a baking sheet.

> **1½ cups walnuts**

Bake the nuts until toasted and fragrant, 7 to 12 minutes. Remove from oven; let cool about 15 minutes. Set aside and make sure to reserve ¼ cup walnuts for the final garnish.

Make the crust. Combine the following ingredients in a food processor. Process the mixture until it is finely ground and begins to clump, about 30 seconds. Stop and scrape down the sides of the bowl if needed. Add an additional teaspoon or 2 of water if it does not stick together when pinched.

> **1¼ cups of the roasted walnuts**
> **6 pitted Medjool dates, each cut into a few pieces**
> **½ cup old fashioned oats**
> **3 tablespoons oat flour**
> **2 teaspoons chia seeds, ground in a small blender, coffee grinder, or spice grinder (see additional ground chia seeds needed in the caramel filling)**
> **2 teaspoons vanilla extract or vanilla powder**
> **2 teaspoons water**
> **⅛ teaspoon salt (or to taste)**

Press the mixture evenly into the bottom of your pan and about 1 inch up the sides.

Bake the crust until the edges are a light golden brown, 8 to 12 minutes. Transfer to a wire rack and, while it's warm, run a thin, small knife around the edge to separate the crust from the pan. Let the crust cool for at least 20 minutes.

(Continued on page 246)

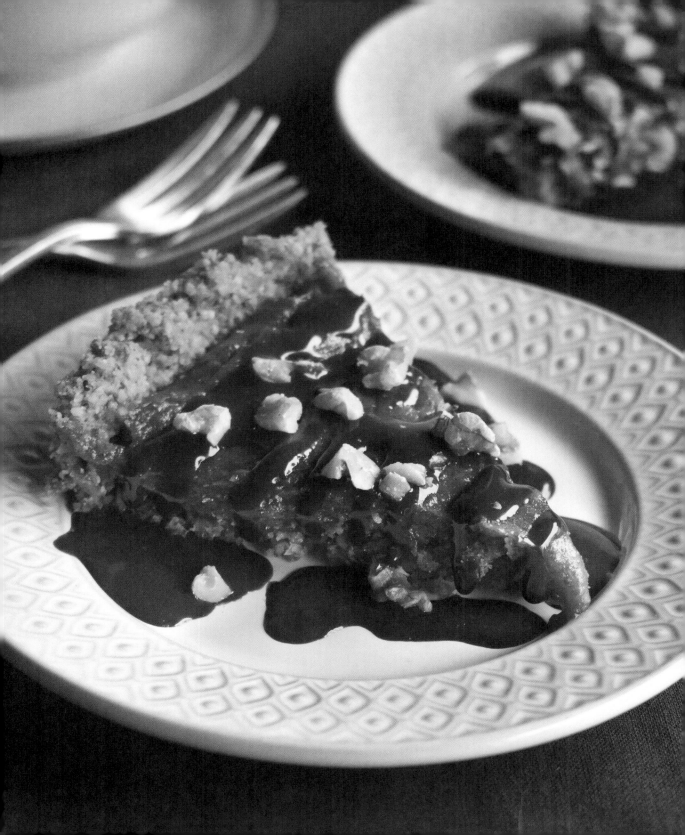

Make the caramel filling. Blend the following ingredients together in a full-size blender until smooth. (Note that a small blender does not work well for this job.)

- **15 Medjool dates**
- **⅓ cup warm water**
- **3 tablespoons almond butter**
- **1 tablespoon vanilla extract or vanilla powder**
- **1½ teaspoons chia seeds, ground in a small blender, coffee grinder, or spice grinder**
- **Pinch of salt (optional)**

Spread the mixture evenly over the crust. Chill in the refrigerator for at least 3 to 4 hours to set.

For serving, unhinge the springform pan and remove the outside rim. Cut slices of the tart and plate them. Drizzle chocolate sauce on the slices and garnish with roasted walnuts.

- **Everywhere All-at-Once Chocolate Sauce (page 263)**
- **¼ cup roasted walnuts, chopped**

The tart will keep, covered and refrigerated, for 3 to 4 days. It does not freeze well.

Apple Crisp with Dates and Oats

Makes 8 servings

Fruit crisps have been one of my favorite desserts since I had my first bite of a crisp around age twenty. The key to this recipe is baking the apples by themselves to soften them up, then continuing to bake them with the topping. The result is a base of sweet baked apples slices with a crumbly streusel on top. Granny Smith apples also work (as do other fruits like berries, peaches, and pears), but the anthocyanin compounds in the peels of red apples provide the best anti-inflammatory boost.

Preheat the oven to 375°F. Make in an 11 × 8-inch baking dish or deep-dish pie pan.

Prepare the apples. Core the apples. Thinly slice them into a large bowl (or cut them into chunks if you prefer).

> 2½–3 pounds red apples, unpeeled (I recommend a combination of Honeycrisp, Gala, Braeburn, and/or Pink Lady)

Toss the apples together with the flour.

> 2 tablespoons oat flour or whole wheat pastry flour

Add the following ingredients to the bowl of floured apples and gently stir until all apples are coated.

> ½ cup maple syrup
> 2 tablespoons freshly squeezed lemon juice
> 1 teaspoon cinnamon
> 1 teaspoon vanilla extract or vanilla powder
> ¼ teaspoon nutmeg
> ¼ teaspoon ginger powder

Bake the apples. Spoon the mixture into your baking dish. Cover with foil and bake for a total of 45 minutes, gently stirring the apples and redistributing after 25 minutes. While the apples are baking, make the topping.

Make the topping. Chop the dates and flour in a food processor until the dates are about the size of peas.

> 8 Medjool dates, each cut into 3–4 pieces (about 1 cup)
> ½ cup oat flour or whole wheat pastry flour

(Continued on page 249)

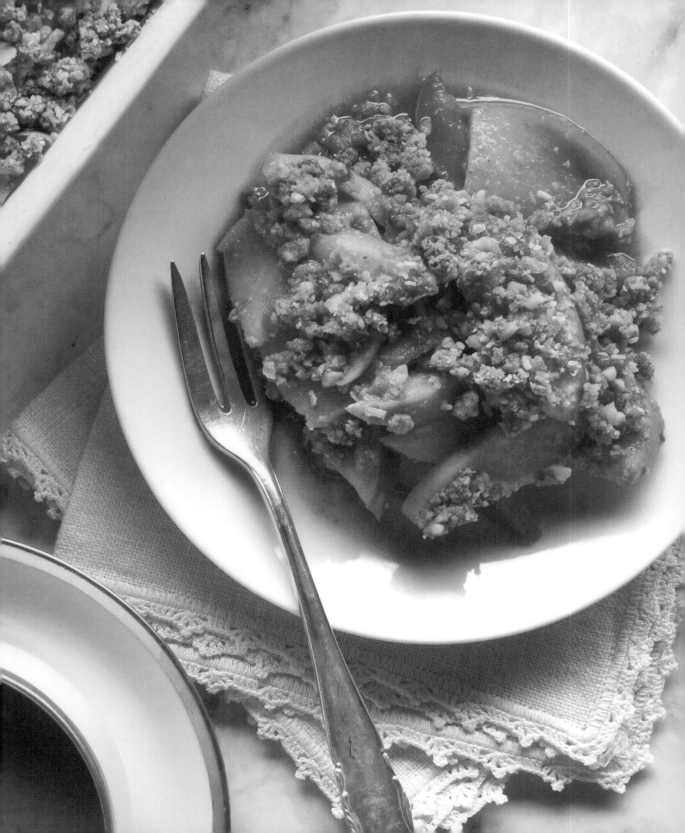

Add in the following ingredients and pulse to combine them with the dates.

¼ **cup quick cooking or old fashioned oats**
¼ **cup unsweetened flaked or shredded coconut**
¼ **cup cashew or almond butter**
⅛ **teaspoon salt (optional)**

The mixture should hold together enough to make clumps. If it's too dry, add in a tablespoon of water at a time until you reach a clump consistency.

Stir in the almonds and set the topping aside until the apples have baked.

¼ **cup slivered almonds**

Assemble and bake (again). Remove the baked apples from the oven. Gently stir and redistribute the apples again, then spread the topping on the apples, pressing down on the topping a bit. Bake the crisp for 25 to 30 minutes, uncovered, or until the filling is bubbly and the topping is golden (be careful, because it can burn quickly). Allow the crisp to cool at least 10 to 15 minutes before serving.

Serve with Ginger-Infused Cream Topping or other topping, if desired.

Ginger-Infused Cream Topping (page 264)

The crisp will be best on the first day—after that, the topping will not be as crisp, but it will still be delicious. It will keep in the refrigerator for 3 to 4 days. It does not freeze well.

No-Bake Cherry Cookie Balls

Makes 20–24 balls

I love having a container of these no-bake cookie balls in my fridge. Just one of them is enough to satisfy a sudden craving for something sweet. This recipe requires less cleanup than most. No mixing bowls or baking pans. Just a food processor. Chewy and filling, the balls get their sweetness from dates and dried cherries and their crunch from roasted seeds. This recipe would be great to make with kids.

Place the following ingredients in a food processor and process until the mixture starts to clump. If it doesn't clump, add more water, a teaspoon at a time.

1⅓ cups Medjool dates
⅔ cup quick or old fashioned uncooked oats
½ cup slivered, sliced, or chopped almonds, best if roasted
2 tablespoons flaxseed meal
1 tablespoon maple syrup
1 teaspoon water
½ teaspoon cinnamon
½ teaspoon vanilla extract or vanilla powder

Add in the following ingredients and pulse until just mixed in.

3 tablespoons roasted and salted/unsalted sunflower seeds or other roasted nuts
3 tablespoon dried cherries, roughly chopped

With your hands, roll about a tablespoon of mixture into a tight ball and set it in a container with a lid. Repeat with the remaining mixture. Store in a covered container and refrigerate for several hours until chilled. The cookie balls will last 1 to 2 weeks in the refrigerator and they freeze well.

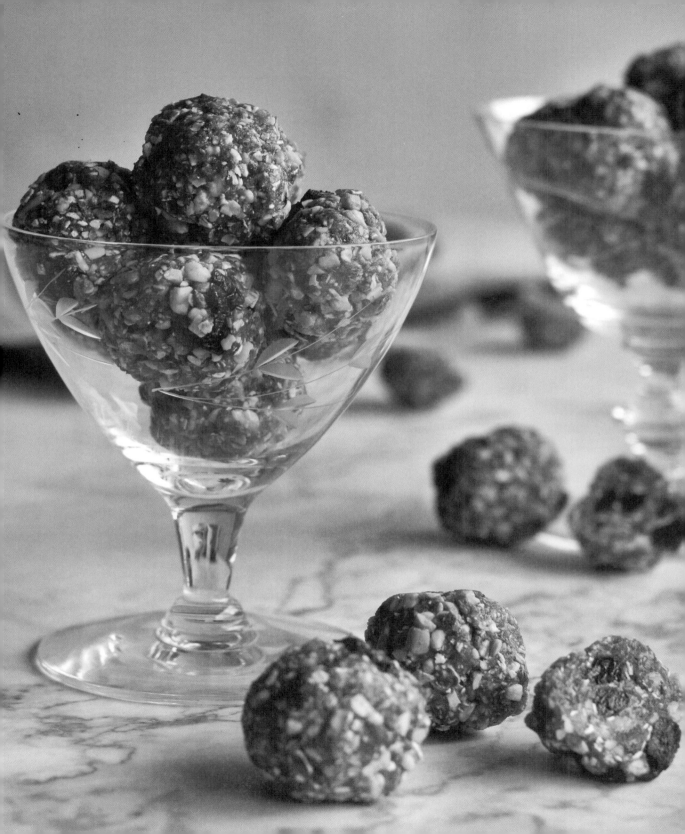

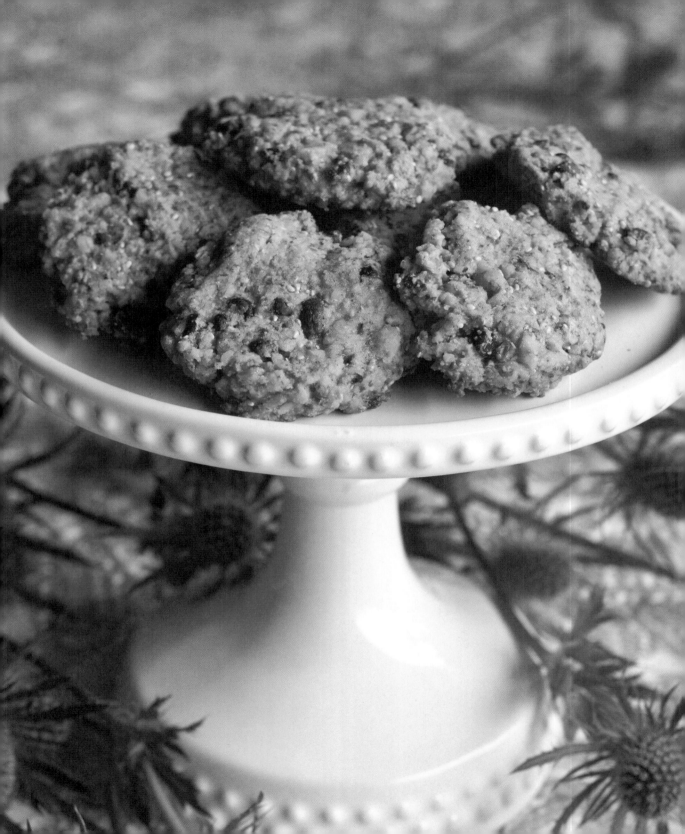

Walnut Cocoa Nib Cookies

Makes 15–20 cookies

These gems remind me of the nut-based cookies my German grandmother sent to us every Christmas—we fought over the exotic treats, each of us declaring loudly which one was our favorite. Walnuts make these cookies moist and complex—what a bonus that they are high in omega-3, a natural inflammation fighter. You can substitute dried fruit for the cocoa nibs, but if you haven't had cocoa nibs before, you might want to try them here—nibs are crushed pieces of roasted cocoa beans without added sugar or fat.

Preheat the oven to 350°F. Line two sheet pans with parchment paper or silicone mats.

Pulse the walnuts in a food processor until they are in small pieces. You can also use a handheld grinder.

2 cups walnuts

In a medium mixing bowl, add the following ingredients and stir well.

The walnuts
½ cup oat flour
⅓ cup maple syrup
¼ cup cocoa nibs, raisins, dried cranberries, dried cherries, or other dried fruit
3 tablespoons flaxseed meal
2 tablespoons white or black chia seeds
2 teaspoons vanilla extract or vanilla powder
⅛ teaspoon salt (or to taste)

Use a 1½-tablespoon cookie scoop or spoon to drop mounds of dough onto the sheet pans. Flatten the cookies with your hand, a fork, or the bottom of a glass (moistened if needed to prevent sticking). Bake the cookies for 10 to 12 minutes or until golden brown—it's important for them not to burn to a dark brown.

Let the cookies cool on the pans. They are ready to eat as soon as you can handle them, or they can be stored in an airtight container at room temperature for several days. They freeze well.

Orange-Cherry Cardamom Bars

Makes 1 (8 × 8-inch) pan of bars

The inspiration for these bars came from the Mayan Wonder Bars at Portland's Dragonfly Coffee House. I've tinkered my way to healthy, chewy, moist, seed-filled bars that have a beguiling combination of flavors. Toasting the seeds, nuts, and quinoa separately would take quite a while, so I came up with a method for staggering their starting times. These bars are dense, not cake-like. The various flavors emerge the longer you chew.

Preheat the oven to 350°F. Line an 8 × 8-inch baking pan with parchment paper.

Roast the quinoa, nuts, and seeds. Spread the following ingredients on a 13 × 9-inch or 16 × 12-inch pan. Bake them in the oven for 7 minutes.

⅓ cup raw pumpkin seeds
¼ cup uncooked quinoa

Remove the pan from the oven and add the following ingredients. Bake for another 7 minutes. Everything should be aromatic and starting to brown. Set aside.

¼ cup raw sunflower seeds
¼ cup raw walnuts, pecans, cashews, or macadamia nuts, chopped
⅛ cup hemp or sesame seeds

Make the date/chia paste. Grind the chia seeds in a small blender until powdery.

1½ tablespoons chia seeds

Add in the following ingredients and blend again until smooth.

⅔ cup warm water
4–5 Medjool dates, cut into a few pieces each (about ½ cup)

Put it all together and bake. In a medium bowl, stir together the following ingredients until smooth.

The date/chia paste
Zest from 2 oranges
¾ cup almond butter (almond *butter*, not *flour*)
½ cup whole wheat pastry flour or gluten-free flour
¼ cup date syrup or maple syrup

(Continued on page 256)

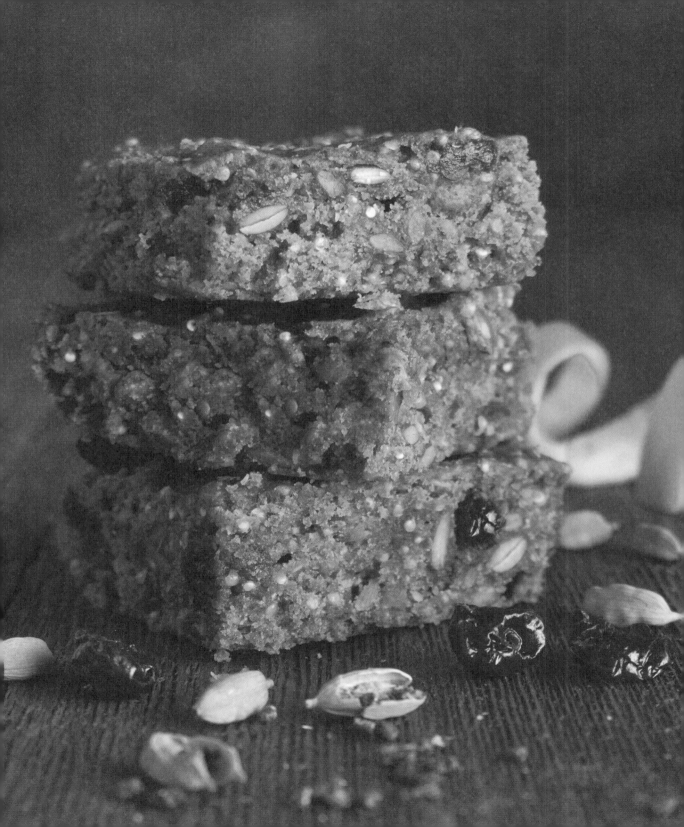

2 teaspoons cardamom powder

1 teaspoon baking powder

½ teaspoon cinnamon

Add in the following ingredients and stir again.

The roasted quinoa, nuts, and seeds

½ cup dried cherries or other dried fruit of choice, chopped

Spread the mixture in the baking pan and bake for 25 to 30 minutes until the bars are golden brown and the sides are a darker shade of brown. Allow them to cool completely, then refrigerate them. Store the bars in the refrigerator, where they will keep for about a week. They can be frozen.

Rice Pudding with Cardamom and Cinnamon

Makes 4 servings

My pressure-cooking classes are among my most popular, and rice pudding is a great dessert to make in the pressure cooker. I set myself the goal of creating a delicious pudding made with brown rice instead of white and without refined sugar. This version is rich and creamy, studded with dried fruit, and laced with cinnamon and cardamom, two of my favorite spices and both loaded with healthy antioxidants. Rice pudding this healthy makes a great breakfast, too.

Pressure cooker directions. Add the water and rice to an electric pressure cooker. Lock the lid. Move the knob to "Sealing." Use the "High," "Pressure Cook," "Multigrain," or "Manual" mode and set for 22 minutes. Wait for 10 minutes after the pressure cooker is done, then move the knob to "Venting" and release the remaining steam before opening the lid.

> **1 cup uncooked brown rice (I prefer short-grain brown rice for this dessert), rinsed**
> **1⅓ cups water**

Meanwhile, make the cashew milk. Soak the cashews in water for 2 hours or pour boiling water over them, cover, let them soak for about 20 minutes, then drain them.

> **⅓ cup raw cashews**

Put the cashews and water in a blender. Blend on high for 30 seconds or longer, until the cashews are dissolved.

> **1¾ cups water**

Finish the pudding. Once you have unlocked the lid, press the "Sauté" button on the pressure cooker. Add the following ingredients to the pressure cooker pot and stir with the cooked rice.

> **The cashew milk**
> **3 tablespoons maple syrup**
> **1 teaspoon vanilla extract or vanilla powder**
> **½ teaspoon cardamom**
> **¼ teaspoon cinnamon**

(Continued on page 259)

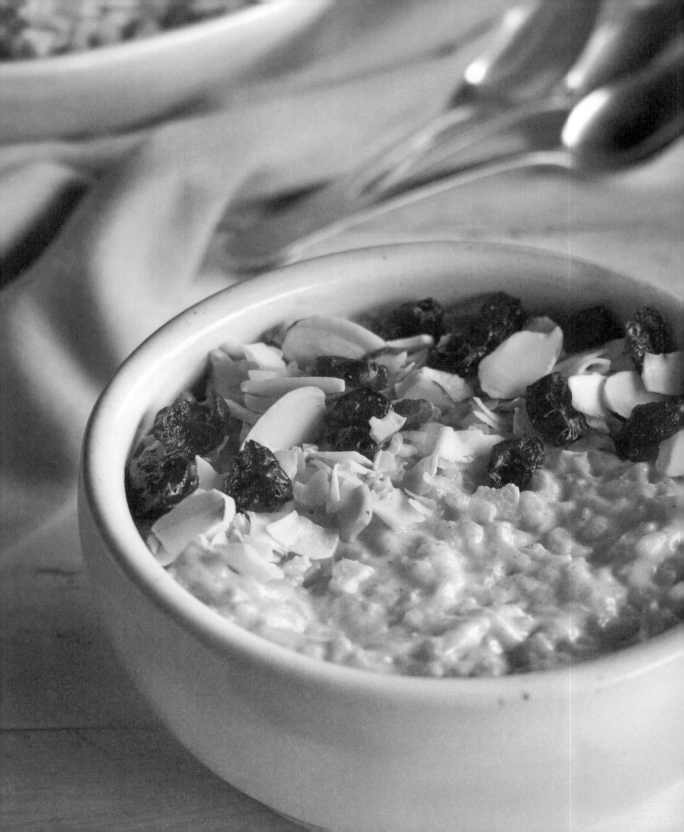

Bring the mixture to a boil in the pot and stir continuously once it is boiling. If your pressure cooker has a low setting for the sauté mode, switch to low, but high works as well (you can turn the cooker off if it gets too hot). Cook and stir for 2 to 3 minutes after the mixture comes to a boil. It should be creamy at this point. Add more water if it is too thick or cook longer if it is too thin (it will also thicken as it cools). Once the mixture is creamy, remove the pot from the pressure cooker (with oven mitts) to avoid further cooking. Stir in the dried fruit.

⅓ cup dried cherries, raisins, or other dried fruit

Stovetop directions. Cook the brown rice according to package directions, or use the Whole Grains Cooking Guide on page 43. When the rice is done, stir in the cashew milk, maple syrup, vanilla, cardamom, and cinnamon. Bring the mixture to a boil and stir continuously once it boils. Cook and stir for 2 to 3 minutes, at which point it should be creamy. Add more water if it is too thick, or cook longer if it is too thin. Once the mixture is creamy, remove the pot from the stove to avoid further cooking. Follow the above instructions for adding the dried fruit.

Let the pudding sit for at least 5 minutes to cool. You can serve it immediately or store it in the refrigerator. If you store it in the fridge, it will likely need more milk or water when you eat it later. The pudding will last in the refrigerator for 4 to 5 days. It does not freeze well.

You can eat your pudding cold or warm and top with one or more of the following ingredients.

Additional dried fruit
Diced fresh fruit such as mango or peach
Roasted nuts such as walnuts, pistachios, or sliced almonds
Toasted or raw shredded coconut
Everywhere All-at-Once Chocolate Sauce (page 263)
Cacao nibs

Mascarpone Cheese with Berries

Makes about 2 cups

Mascarpone (pronounced mass-car-POH-nay) cheese is best known as a component of tiramisu, a traditional Italian dessert made with ladyfingers, coffee, amaretto, and chocolate shavings. This soft cheese is made from heavy cream and tastes similar to cream cheese and crème fraîche, but with a little more sweetness. This plant-based version achieves its rich, silky texture from cashews, which are blended until completely dissolved. I suggest serving this mascarpone on berries, but it can be used as a topping for all sorts of desserts as well as in pasta dishes.

Soak the cashews. Soak the cashews in water for 2 hours or pour boiling water over them, cover, let them soak for about 20 minutes, then drain them.

2 cups raw cashews

Make the mascarpone. Put the following ingredients in a blender. Blend on high for 30 seconds or more, until the cashews are dissolved and the mixture is very smooth.

The soaked and drained cashews
⅔ cup water
¼ cup maple syrup
2 tablespoons freshly squeezed lemon juice
1 teaspoon nutritional yeast
1 teaspoon lemon zest
1 teaspoon white miso

Transfer to an airtight plastic or glass container. Chill for several hours to let it thicken. It will last about a week in the fridge and can also be frozen (you may need to blend it after thawing to restore the texture).

Serve with berries or blend it with berries as a topping for fruit or cake.

Berries of choice

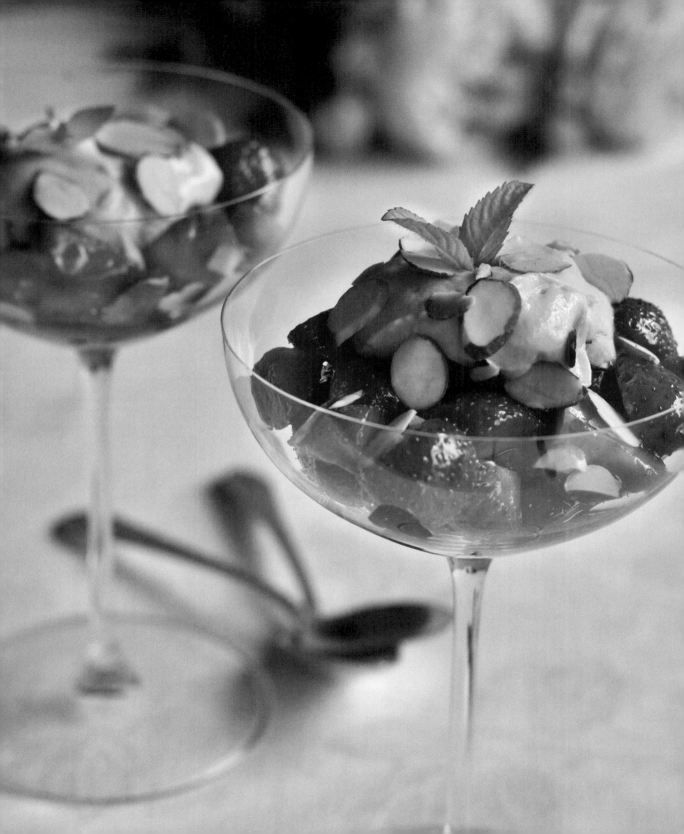

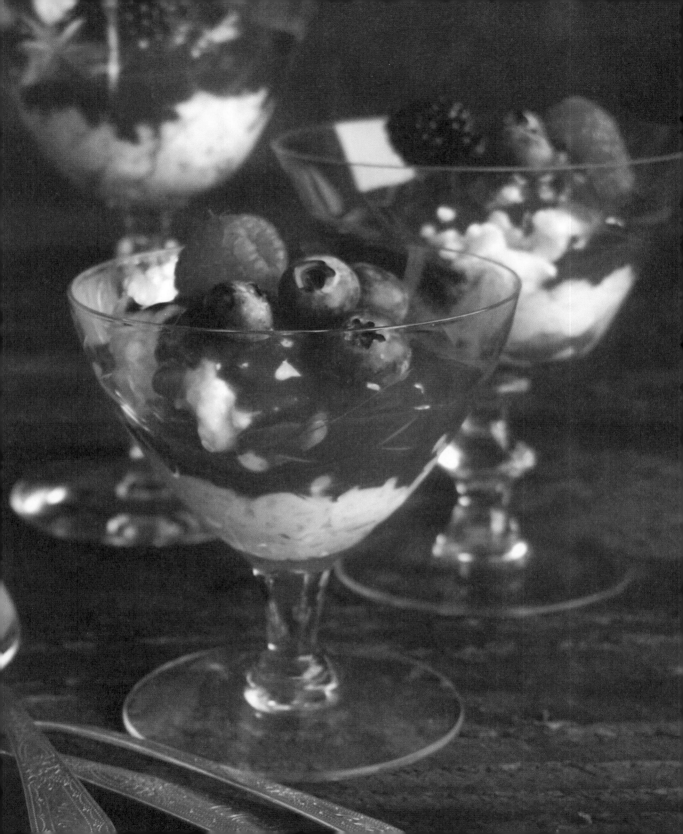

Everywhere All-at-Once Chocolate Sauce

Makes about 1 cup

A great chocolate sauce is like the perfect little black dress—it goes with everything and is perfect for any occasion. As a bonus, this sauce is very easy to make. It goes well on cakes, tarts, nice cream, puddings, pancakes, waffles, or as a dip for fruit. If you have a tree nut allergy, you could substitute sunflower seed butter, pumpkin seed butter, or peanut butter for the almond butter. You can buy date syrup or you can make your own.

Blend the following ingredients together in a small or large blender or with a stick (immersion) blender until smooth.

- ⅔ cup **date syrup**
- ¼ cup **almond butter**
- ¼ cup **water**
- 3 tablespoons **cocoa powder**
- 4 teaspoons **vanilla extract or vanilla powder**

The chocolate sauce is ready to use. It will last 1 to 2 weeks in the refrigerator—you may need to stir in more water if it gets too thick. It can be frozen.

Ginger-Infused Cream Topping

Makes about 2 cups

My quest for a healthy non-coconut topping has been a long one. Coconut cream contains a lot of saturated fat. Cashews are a good alternative, but I wanted a cream that would be lighter than an all-cashew cream. Enter tofu. It's lighter in fat and calories than cashews, and using a combination of tofu and cashews works wonderfully. The type of tofu determines the final consistency of the this topping, so choose your tofu wisely. The bonus with this cream is a subtle hint of ginger (or, alternatively, orange or lemon). This versatile cream goes with almost any dessert.

Soak the cashews. Soak the cashews in water for 2 hours or pour boiling water over them, cover, let them soak for about 20 minutes, then drain them.

⅔ **cup raw cashews**

Make the cream. Place the following ingredients in a blender. Blend on high until the cashews are dissolved and the mixture is completely smooth.

The soaked and drained cashews
1⅓ cups tofu (extra firm and firm tofu yield a spoonable cream; silken tofu yields a pourable cream)
⅓ **cup maple syrup**
2 teaspoons freshly squeezed lemon juice
2 teaspoons vanilla extract or vanilla powder
2 teaspoons fresh ginger, finely chopped, or 1 teaspoon lemon or orange zest
1 teaspoon white miso (optional, but it adds depth of flavor)

Transfer the mixture to an airtight container and refrigerate for several hours so that it chills and thickens. The cream will last 4 to 5 days in the refrigerator. It can be frozen; you may need to reblend it to restore the texture.

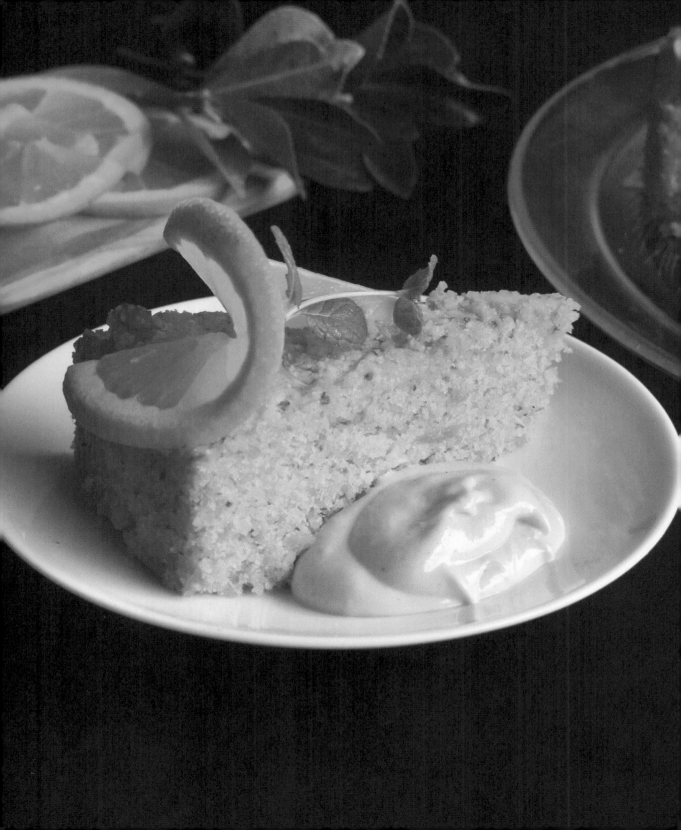

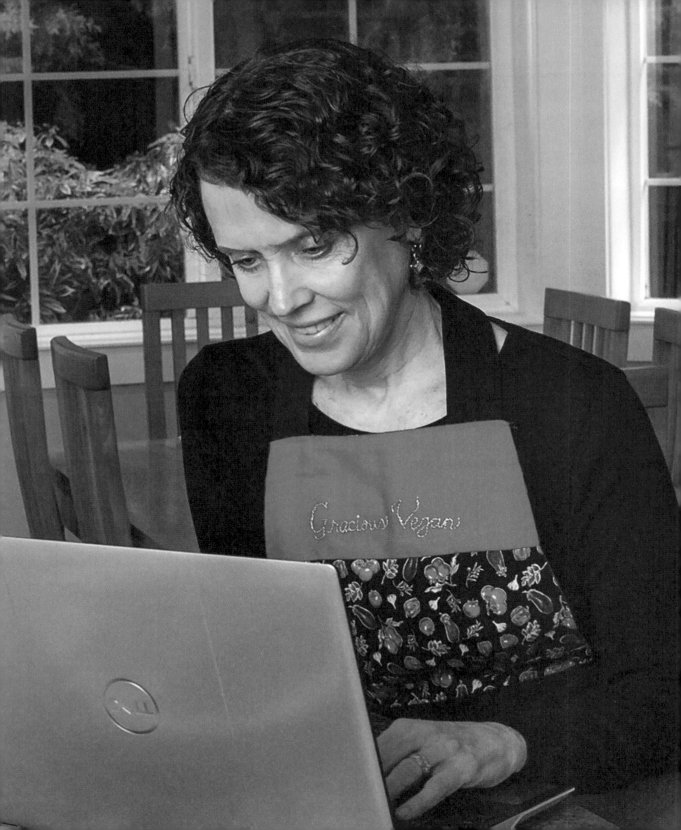

Resources and Deep Dives

I've always loved learning, which must be why I stayed in school until I got a PhD. As I conducted the research for this book and dug deep into inflammation and a plant-based anti-inflammatory diet, I found a world of excellent resources, even beyond what I already knew. For your benefit, I've whittled down my recommendations to the best of the best. I hope you'll find them as useful as I have.

Inflammation
Monica Aggarwal and Jyothi Rao, *Body on Fire: How Inflammation Triggers Chronic Illness and the Tools We Have to Fight It*

This book by two physicians explains inflammation and its causes in clear, approachable language. Dr. Aggarwal tells of her own route to completely calming the pain and swelling of rheumatoid arthritis through diet and lifestyle changes. The authors offer a great deal of practical advice for implementing science-supported ways to lower inflammation.

Shilpa Ravella, *A Silent Fire: The Story of Inflammation, Diet, and Disease*

I read Shilpa Ravella's book when I was supposed to be reading a light fiction book for a book club. This fascinating history of the discovery of the immune response and inflammation was a page-turner I couldn't put down! The book-club novel sat on the side table unread. Dr. Ravella explains inflammation in understandable terms and reports on the types of foods and lifestyle changes that have been shown to lower inflammation. But the drama of scientific discovery over a century and a half is what makes it worth the read.

Brooke Goldner, MD: goodbyelupus.com

Rooted in Dr. Goldner's own experience as a former lupus sufferer, this site offers free online classes aimed to help those who have autoimmune diseases. Based on her own healing journey and expertise as a doctor, she provides practical advice on how to get healthy and lower your autoimmune-induced suffering.

Plant-Based Nutritional Information
NutritionFacts.org

I've been a volunteer writer and reviewer for this organization for over eight years now because I believe in its science-rooted approach and its mission to generously share solid scientific information with the public. Founder Dr. Michael Greger and his expert team distill the results of peer-reviewed nutritional studies into explanatory videos and blogs that are free for anyone to view. Dr. Greger's companion books—*How Not to Die*, *How Not to Diet* and *How Not to Age*—are must-reads to understand the science supporting a plant-based approach to eating and thriving.

Physicians' Committee on Responsible Medicine (PCRM): pcrm.org

PCRM is an advocacy organization that promotes a plant-based diet, preventive medicine, and alternatives to animal research. They provide tools for transitioning to a plant-based diet and have developed excellent handouts about many different health conditions that can be addressed with diet. They've created nutritional education tools for clinicians as well as conducted their own research studies where they've seen gaps. Their "Health Topics" section features excellent summaries on a variety of topics.

Dr. Joel Fuhrman: drfuhrman.com

Known for advocating a nutrient-dense or "nutritarian" diet and daily "G-BOMBS" (greens, berries, onions, mushrooms, beans, and seeds), Dr. Fuhrman provides a wealth of information about a healthy plant-based diet, including summaries of the science behind his dietary recommendations and practical advice on the best types of foods to eat every day. His books *Eat to Live*, *Super Immunity*, *The End of Dieting*, and *The End of Heart Disease* are excellent. Dr. Fuhrman sells a line of products and membership in his community, but you don't have to purchase anything to get a lot of information from his site.

Plant-Based Cooking, Lifestyle, and Learning
Chef AJ: youtube.com/c/CHEFAJ

Chef AJ—a chef, cookbook author, teacher, and motivational speaker in her own right—hosts a daily interview show with doctors, psychologists, dieticians, chefs, entrepreneurs, and other healthy vegan professionals. I've had the pleasure of being her guest several times. She has a special mission to help those struggling with weight management and frequently hosts experts on food addiction and other weight issues. The interviews and demos are enjoyable to watch. I always learn something.

Forks Over Knives: forksoverknives.com

This packed website got its start in the wake of the popular documentary *Forks Over Knives*, which was based on Dr. T. Colin Campbell's seminal book, *The China Project*. The website offers hundreds of free recipes, meal ideas, and resources. It also offers two companion apps: Forks Plant-Based Recipes and Forks Meal Planner, available for free with in-app purchase options or at a low one-time price.

Food Revolution Network: foodrevolution.org

Founded by John and Ocean Robbins, this organization is best known for its annual Food Revolution Summits, an online docuseries featuring interviews with top nutritional experts. The Summits are in-depth, engaging, and well-produced. They are free for a limited time when they premiere, or you can purchase a package for lifetime access.

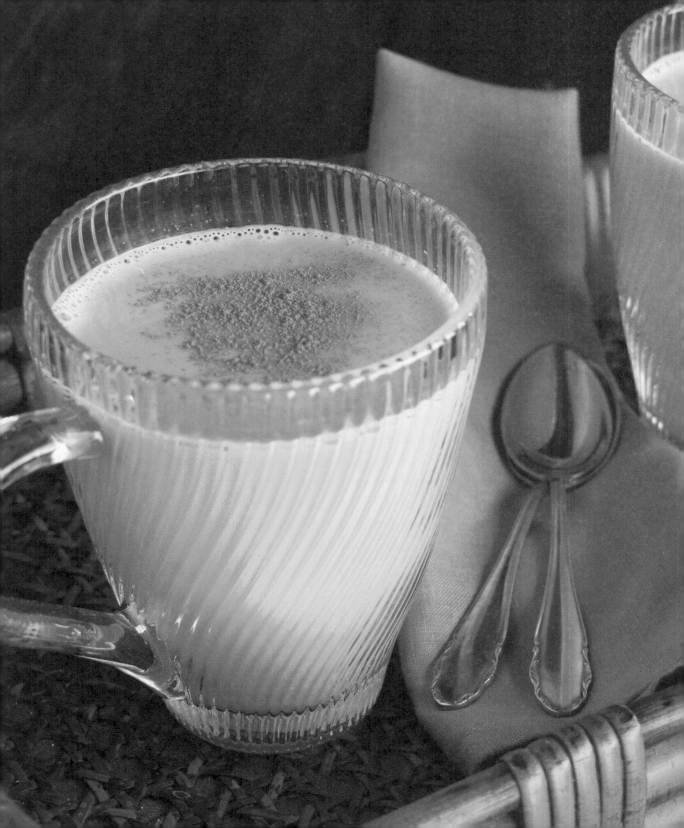

Acknowledgments

I owe so much to so many people for their help and support on this project.

Chef AJ, thank you for taking a chance on an unknown blogger and cooking instructor who emailed you out of the blue. You let me guest on your YouTube show, invited me back, and encouraged me to write a cookbook. That boost of confidence got this project started.

Ashley Madden, I'm so grateful to you for sharing your publishing experience with me and helping me start my navigation toward this goal.

To my recipe testers—Susan Hanson, Cassandra Hill, Steven Kaufman, Brenda Parulski, Anne Walther, and Lori Watts—thanks so, so much for sticking with me these many months. You did a heck of a lot of work and gave me such helpful feedback. My recipes got better because of your work, and your faith in me has kept me going.

Jon Deshler, photography lessons with you took me from a self-taught amateur stuck in a rut to a photographer who is in much more control of the dynamic elements that make an arresting food photo. Your eagle eye for details and your emphasis on process helped me immensely.

Julia Gagne, thank you for the lovely handmade bowls you gave me for this project. They proved to be perfect vessels for soups, hot cereals, and puddings. I loved using them in my photos.

Dr. Kristi Funk, Colleen Kelleher, and Brenda Davis, RD, thank you for your thoughtful reviews of selected chapters. Your comments helped me improve the manuscript.

Editor Nicole Mele and the Skyhorse team, you've been wonderful partners in getting this book from draft to bookshelf. Thank you for all the care and creativity you've put into it and for taking a chance on this first-timer.

To my friends, students, and family who have encouraged me along this path, I appreciate you more than I can say. Your kind words about my cooking, photos, and ideas have strengthened me and helped me better define what I bring to the culinary world.

Mom, I wish you were here to see this. The warm, safe, peaceful home you created allowed me to start learning and growing into the person I am today. You showed that loving a family through food doesn't mean making an extravagant meal every now and then, but providing healthy, tasty food meal by meal, seven days a week. You are still my original hero.

Lori Watts, I couldn't ask for a better sister. Thanks especially for posing as the "hands" on all those cold winter afternoons in my garage studio. Your interest, support, and cheering have helped me so much.

Doug Fiero, what would I have done without your encouragement, patience, and modeling of the "art life"? You've adapted to my second career with grace and understanding, including all the Zoom classes from the kitchen that force you into other parts of the house. Your read-throughs and edits have lifted the quality of my writing. Thank you for being my biggest fan.

Metric Conversions

If you're accustomed to using metric measurements, use these handy charts to convert the imperial measurements used in this book.

Weight (Dry Ingredients)

1 oz		30 g
4 oz	¼ lb	120 g
8 oz	½ lb	240 g
12 oz	¾ lb	360 g
16 oz	1 lb	480 g
32 oz	2 lb	960 g

Oven Temperatures

Fahrenheit	Celsius	Gas Mark
225°	110°	¼
250°	120°	½
275°	140°	1
300°	150°	2
325°	160°	3
350°	180°	4
375°	190°	5
400°	200°	6
425°	220°	7
450°	230°	8

Volume (Liquid Ingredients)

½ tsp.		2 ml
1 tsp.		5 ml
1 Tbsp.	½ fl oz	15 ml
2 Tbsp.	1 fl oz	30 ml
¼ cup	2 fl oz	60 ml
⅓ cup	3 fl oz	80 ml
½ cup	4 fl oz	120 ml
⅔ cup	5 fl oz	160 ml
¾ cup	6 fl oz	180 ml
1 cup	8 fl oz	240 ml
1 pt	16 fl oz	480 ml
1 qt	32 fl oz	960 ml

Length

¼ in	6 mm
½ in	13 mm
¾ in	19 mm
1 in	25 mm
6 in	15 cm
12 in	30 cm

Index

The Plant-Based Anti-Inflammatory Cookbook

281
Index